Nitroglycerin 7

Nitroglycerin 7

Progress in therapy

Seventh Hamburg Symposium

Editor
P. G. Hugenholtz

Walter de Gruyter
Berlin · New York 1991

This book contains 33 figures and 4 tables.

Library of Congress Cataloging-in-Publication Data

Hamburger Symposium (7th : 1990)
Nitroglycerin 7 : progress in therapy / Seventh Hamburg Symposium ; editor. P. G. Hugenholtz.
p. cm.
Symposium held on Nov. 24, 1990.
ISBN 3-11-013396-2
1. Nitroglycerin – Congresses. 2. Myocardial infarction – Chemotherapy – Congresses. I. Hugenholtz. P. G. II. Title. III. Title: Nitroglycerin seven.
[DNLM; 1. Angina. Pectoris – drug therapy – congresses.
2. Trinitrate – therapeutic use – congresses. WG 298 H199n 1990] RC684.N65H36 1991
616.1'22061 – dc20
DNLM/DLC 91-28638
for Library of Congress
CIP

Die Deutsche Bibliothek – CIP-Einheitsaufnahme

Nitroglycerin 7 : progress in therapy / Seventh Hamburg Symposium, [November 24, 1990]. Ed. P. G. Hugenholtz. – Berlin ; New York : de Gruyter, 1991
Dt. Ausg. u.d.T.: Nitroglycerin VII
ISBN 3-11-013396-2
NE: Hugenholtz, Paul G. [Hrsg.]; Hamburger Nitroglycerin-Symposion <7, 1990>

Medical science is constantly developing. Research and clinical experience expand our knowledge, especially with regard to treatment and medication. For dosages and applications mentioned in this work, the reader may rely on the authors, editors and publisher having taken great pains to ensure that these indications reflect the standard of knowledge at the time this work was completed.
Nevertheless, all users are requested to check the package leaflet of the medication, in order to determine for themselves whether the recommentations given for the dosages or the likely contraindications differ from those given in this book. This is especially true for medication which is seldom used or has recently been put on the market and for medication whose application has been restricted by the German Ministry of Health.
The quotation of registered names, trade names, trade marks, etc. in this copy does not imply, even in the absence of a specific statement that such names are exempt from laws and regulations protecting trade marks, etc. and therefore free for general use.
Typesetting: Arthur Collignon GmbH, Berlin. – Printing: Gerike GmbH, Berlin. – Binding: Dieter Mikolai, Berlin. – Printed in Germany.

Contents

Editor

Prof. Dr. P. G. Hugenholtz

President of SOCAR S.A.
Case Postale 410
CH-1260 Nyon (VD)

List of Contributors

Prof. Dr. W.-D. Bussmann

Klinikum der
Johann-Wolfgang-Goethe-Universität
Zentrum der Inneren Medizin
Abteilung für Kardiologie
Theodor-Stern-Kai 7
D-6000 Frankfurt 70
Deutschland

Prof. Dr. E. I. Chazov

USSR Cardiology Research Centre
Cherepkovskaja ul. 15
Moskau 121 500
UdSSR

Prof. Dr. R. Hetzer

Abteilung für Herzchirurgie
Deutsches Herzzentrum Berlin
Augustenburger Platz 1
D-1000 Berlin 65
Deutschland

Prof. Dr. B. I. Jugdutt

Department of Medicine
Division of Cardiology
University of Alberta
Edmonton, Alberta
Kanada

Dr. M. Kriegmair	Urologische Klinik und Poliklinik Ludwig-Maximilians-Universität Klinikum Großhadern Marchianinistraße 15 D-8000 München 70 Deutschland
Prof. Dr. H.-P. Nast	Innere Medizinische Abteilung Ketteler-Krankenhaus Lichtplattenweg 85 D-6050 Offenbach Deutschland
Prof. Dr. E. Noack	Institut für Pharmakologie Heinrich-Heine-Universität Moorenstraße 5 D-4000 Düsseldorf Deutschland
Prof. Dr. M. O'Rourke	Medical Professorial Unit University of New South Wales St. Vincent's Hospital Sydney 2010 Australien
Priv. Doz. Dr. Staritz	I. Medizinische Klinik und Poliklinik Johannes-Gutenberg-Universität Langenbeckstraße 1 D-6500 Mainz Deutschland
Prof. Dr. H. J. C. Swan	University of California School of Medicine 1075 Wallace Ridge Beverly Hills CA. 90210 USA

Introduction

P. G. Hugenholtz

It is perhaps amazing that at this VIIth Hamburger Nitroglycerin-Symposium there will still be new things to say about this drug that is celebrating its 100th birthday.

There are three main reasons for this observation.

Firstly, it remains a remarkably effective compound, particularly in its various dosages and formulations to "relieve" the heart. As Swan explains in this symposium, relative to other drugs, nitrate therapy has kept its place or, of cost-effectiveness is a factor to go by, is gaining.

Secondly, the elucidation of the endothelin story as well as the understanding and management of the tolerance issue has now made the drug once more respectable. Contributions by Noack and O'Rourke prove this.

Thirdly, other systems than the cardio-vascular have benefitted from its powerful dilating action. Examples in this congress are the contributions by Hofstetter and Staritz. Finally, even in established indications such as acute myocardial infarction and hypertensive crisis new information will be presented by Bussmann and Nast.

Then of course there are other reasons to be together, such as the authoritative review of the cardiac transplanation programme by Hetzer, the recent information by Jugdutt from Canada on the multicentre study for myocardial preservation, and finally a direct inside view of the treatment of patients in the USSR given by Chazov.

This, coupled with the intense competition for the Nitrolingual prize by Pohl-Boskamp, makes for a delightful programme which will stimulate all those who have travelled to Hamburg for this special weekend.

On behalf of all the chairpersons and the organizers, I bid you a heartly welcome to study this text.

The overriding issue of nitrate tolerance

H. J. C. Swan

Tolerance to the vasodepressor actions of nitroglycerin was described more than a century ago [23], yet its clinical relevance has been a matter of concern for only the past decade. This reflects the dominant prior use of nitroglycerin as a short term intermittent form of treatment for a singular form of symptomatic ischemic heart desease – angina pectoris. Nitrate attenuation or tolerance has become clinically significant with the introduction of "long acting" nitrate compounds and continuous or near continuous delivery systems, including intravenous nitroglycerin and transcutaneous administration of nitroglycerin. An attenuation of response, or the need for a higher dosage of nitrates occurs when a significant level of nitrate exists in the blood (and/or tissues) for a period of approximately 20 or more hours. Cross tolerance develops between different compounds. Thus, a patient receiving Isosorbide Dinitrate for 24 hours will have a reduced dilator response to a single dose of sublingual or intravenous nitroglycerin in comparison to the response prior to the initiation of isosorbide-dinitrate. The development of tolerance is also believed to be dose-related, in that an attenuated or absent response develops more rapidly in the presence of high nitrate dosages than in low.

Yet nitrates represent a cornerstone of cardiovascular drug therapy; in significant part due to the lack of dangerous side effects, and their relative cost – low in terms of the majority of cardiac drugs. But the generalised benefit of this simple drug is limited by the rapid attenuation of it's effect when used in conditions other than the acute anginal attack. A solution to this problem is vitally needed.

The mechanism of nitrate tolerance is unknown. Needleman and colleagues [17] suggested that sulfhydryl groups were removed from vascular smooth muscle receptors by a continuous high level of nitrates, resulting in a deficiency of nitrosothiols. The use of N-acetylcysteine has been proposed to limit the development of nitrate tolerance. However the clinical outcomes of trials based on the use of NAC have not been convincing. It has also been suggested that enhancement of sulfhydryl levels in platelets is in some way related to the anti-aggregant action of nitrates. ACE inhibitors have also been suggested as useful adjuncts in the reduction of nitrate attenuation.

The purpose of this manuscript is to examine the complex interplay between nitrates and other factors responsible for vascular tone; the issue of nitrate tolerance or attenuation; and the possible differences in the mechanisms of action and of tolerance between three common diseases for which nitrates are used: Chronic Ischemic Heart Disease, the Acute Ischemic Syndromes, and Acute and Chronic Heart Failure. Further, with expanding application of nitrate therapy to a variety of clinical conditions, it seems naive to expect the manifestations of tolerance or it's mechanisms to be the same or even similar in nature.

Physiologic actions of nitrates

The basic mechanisms of vascular smooth muscle relaxation due to nitrates have been studied in detail by Ignarro [14], Fung [11], Bassenge [2], and Pohl [22] among others. Nitroglycerin and other nitrates are metabolized in vascular smooth muscle to an end product which is, or closely related to nitric oxide NO. This stimulates guanylate-cyclase resulting in a final common effect of smooth muscle relaxation. Of great interest, but confounding in regard to mechanisms of vasomotion, is the discovery of the functional importance of vascular endothelium [12] – a selective barrier to transfer of substances from the blood stream to vascular smooth muscle, and an elaborator of vasodilator and vasoconstrictor substances. The concept that EDRF and nitric oxide may be one and the same still requires absolute proof. Significant differences exist between the actions of, for example nitroglycerin and sodium nitroprusside, and changes in the presence or absence of disorders of endothelial function prevent a clear cut definition of common metabolic pathways. This will be discussed later.

Chronic stable angina pectoris

The classic clinical application of nitroglycerin and the longer acting nitrates has been in the management of chronic stable angina pectoris. Biologically, this disorder is caused by coronary atheroma of differing composition and of differing degrees of luminal intrusion but, with an intact endothelial surface. It is the latter factor that distinguishes this group of conditions from the unstable or acute coronary syndromes in which ulceration and thrombosis play a vital part. In the presence of obstructive coronary artery disease, myocardial blood flow to a given territory is dependent on the aortic pressure during diastole, the duration of diastole, the intra-vascular pressure downstream to obstruction, intra-myocardial resistance including subendocardial systolic vascular compression and the hematocrit.

The work of Brown [4], and of others have indicated that a concentric fixed coronary stenosis exists in approximately 25% of patients with chronic stable angina. In 75% of patients therefore the stenosis is eccentric and an area of normal smooth muscle is present and, therefore, capable of vasomotion. Brown and colleagues [3], using an objective measurement of minimal diameter, also demonstrated a 20 to 30% increase in diameter in response to nitroglycerin which was maximal in vessels between 1.5 and 2.5 millimeters diameter. Larger vessels (left main) were not responsive to the vasodilator effect of nitrates and calcium channel and alpha blocking drugs had minimal effects. These workers also showed an approximate 20% increase in mild to moderate degrees of coronary stenosis but a 36% increase in stenoses graded between 65 and 85%. This was achieved at sublingual doses of nitroglycerin of 0.4 milligrams. Hence the reduction in stenosis flow resistance is substantial. Bearing in mind that a population of patients with coronary disease will include those with concentric stenosis and patients with calcific stenoses, it is clear that a major potential for nitrate induced vasodilatation exists in a significant proportion of such patients.

Nitroglycerin is known clinically to relieve myocardial ischemia. However, its mechanism in patients with chronic stable angina has been debated over the years. Four factors appear to be germain:

- reduction in afterload by reason of peripheral arterial vasodilatation,
- reduction of preload by reason of peripheral venodilatation,
- alterations in the dynamics of coronary blood flow through the stenotic area either by vasodilatation or alteration in sheer forces: and
- dilatation of collateral coronary blood vessels when developed and possessing a significant component of vascular smooth muscle, or
- a combination of all or several of these factors.

For many years vasodilatation in the epicardial coronary vessels was questioned because coronary sinus blood flow failed to increase in response to nitroglycerin [13]. However reductions in preload and afterload would be expected to result in a more uniform transmural distribution of available coronary blood flow during periods of increased demand – exercise or cardiac pacing – and thus reach a greater degree of myocardial efficiency with elimination of the requirement for increased coronary blood flow. However, even this issue is not in itself simple. Vasomotion in epicardial coronary arteries is also related to the magnitude of flow – greater flow causing epicardial vasodilatation. In non-flow limiting atherosclerosis, in spite of responsiveness to nitroglycerin (non-endothelium dependent vasodilatation) the presence of atherosclerosis results in endothelial cell vasodilator dysfunction.

Unstable angina

Intravenous nitroglycerin infusion has been a significant element in the management of patients with unstable angina pectoris. It is now known that unstable angina is characterized by endothelial ulceration and development of thrombus within the plaque itself and extending partially or completely into the lumen of the coronary artery [7]. Nitrates may act in this regard by their anti-aggregation effect on platelets. They may also act by causing vasodilatation in abnormal areas of the vessel wall. Frequently, physicians will continue intravenous nitroglycerin for several days. It is possible that vasoactive tolerance to nitrates develops, but if the thrombus itself or the platelet components are favorably affected, then a satisfactory response could be present although vascular attenuation was equivalent to other situations.

As pointed out, nitroglycerin is an endothelium independent vasodilator. Indeed, it has been shown that vasodilatation may be greater in vascular segments denuded of endothelium [16]. Whether or not this is due to the presence of an increase in resting vascular tone (by reason of deficiency of naturally occurring EDRF) or enhanced sensitivity to nitrate is currently unknown. Nevertheless this represents a highly interesting potential mechanism for the use of nitrates in the unstable coronary syndromes characterized by endothelial ulceration.

Heart failure

As a group of powerful vasodilators, nitrates have been applied in the management of acute and chronic heart failure. Initially, sodium nitroprusside was effective in the treatment of acute pulmonary edema, and in chronic severe heart failure associated with mitral regurgitation [5]. Several hemodynamic mechanisms are relevant. Sodium nitroprusside is an effective arteriolar vasodilator with a lesser venodilator action. Primary afterload reduction allows for a fall in diastolic ventricular pressure, and coaption of the mitral valve leaflets. A high incidence of unrecognized mitral regurgation is found in patients with acute pulmonary edema. Hence it seems that these effects may be due to the direct vascular action on systemic arterioles. However, Kelly and colleagues [15] found that, following nitroglycerin, a reduction in arterial wave reflection causes an important fall in central aortic pressure, although brachial artery systolic pressure was unchanged. Hence, considerations of afterload based on peripheral pulse data which ignore dynamic impedance are likely to be misleading. In the arterial system, dilatation of conductance vessels (2–4 mm.) will not change total vascular resistance, but will alter reflectance.

But chronic heart failure is a different condition. Changes in total body water, in distribution and in vascular smooth muscle calcium take place over days or weeks. Stimulation of the neurohumoral compensatory mechanisms results in alpha-adrenergic activation and angiotensin-renin-alderosterone production. The normal dominance of vasomotion of the resistance vessels by local metabolic controle is lost or attenuated. Intravascular volumes – largely venous – are increased, with altered venous wall tension. In contrast to the coronary arteries, systemic veins and resistance arteries are free of atherosclerosis. Hence, the mechanisms of tolerance are likely to be different from those relevant to chronic stable angina or unstable angina.

Nitrate tolerance

The criteria for the development of tolerance should be examined from both physiological and clinical aspects. As stated the actions of nitrates on vascular smooth muscle are complex, with a hierarchy of responses so that the coronary arteries and systemic veins are most susceptible to the direct vasodilator action of nitrates and systemic arterioles less so. In addition, vasodilatation in the coronary arteries is maximal in the small vessels and of a lesser degree in large ones. Vascular reactivity is also altered by the presence of atherosclerosis. Finally, endothelial ulceration gives rise to yet another series of abnormaties, including the absence of production of EDRF and absence of dilator response to acetylcholine. Endothelial ulceration can also result in intramural hemorrhage and intramural and intraluminal thrombosis.

Endpoints of clinical evaluation of nitrates and thus for the presence or absence of tolerance have been developed over the years but remain less than satisfactory from both physiological and clinical standpoint. The mechanisms underlying angina pectoris are in themselves complex ranging from alteration in demand with a fixed (atherosclerosis) limitation on supply to a highly labile vasomotive state, as in Prinzmetal's angina or in unstable angina to a mixed form of ischemia, in which both fixed and variable (vasomotive) restriction of flow reserve have to meet a variation in oxygen demand. The commonality in nitrate attenuation does appear to be failure of nitrate induced vasodilatation. However, this might be maximal in relation to coronary and systemic venous tone, yet not matter to the same degree in terms of systemic vascular resistance and other mechanisms pertain.

It is inappropriate to extrapolate data from one clinical situation necessarily to another. Thus the response in patients with effort induced angina may be different from those with emotionally induced or rest angina, different still from patients with unstable angina and certainly highly different from patients with chronic heart failure.

Angina pectoris

In clinical trials a reduction in the incidence of anginal episodes or an increased exercise treadmill time are called for as the appropriate endpoints to determine efficacy. Both of these endpoints are notoriously difficult to control and assess. Even in patients with established severe coronary disease anginal episodes are not seen with absolute regularity, and the duration of exercise may vary. In placebo controlled trials the "run-in" studies (prior to medication or dummy) have demonstrated large variations in exercise tolerance. Holter monitoring should provide interesting information in this regard, since the endpoint incidence is approximately 4 times greater than episodes of symptomatic angina pectoris. Vasodilator or vasoconstrictor responses – reactive hyperemia, cold pressor response – might give further insight into the effects of nitrates and tolerance development. However, at the present time, the United States FDA only regard favorable alterations in the incidence of anginal episodes or significant increases in the duration of exercise as being relevant endpoints.

The majority of trials of efficacy of nitrates and the development of tolerance has involved patients with chronic stable angina pectoris. Parker, Thadani and their colleagues [20, 21, 25] completed a series of studies which established the existence of nitrate tolerance without doubt. After 1–2 weeks of oral ISDN (4 times/day), significant attenuation in magnitude and duration of exercise time to angina was observed and the dose-response relationship was lost. With transcutaneous administration, the positive effect at 2 hours on exercise time to angina was attenuated at 24 hours, and in patients treated for 1–2 weeks the effect was completely absent. Continuous intravenous infusion resulted in abolition of the initial nitrate effect by 24 hours and a blunted response to an additional single sublingual dose of nitroglycerin at the end of 24 hours. Most authorities agree that nitrate tolerance may be near complete if a high nitrate concentration is constant for 24 hours or more. However with intermittent dosage with differing drug concentrations over the 24 hours nitrate attenuation may be only partial.

Bassan [1] studied a group of patients with stable exertional angina who had demonstrated increased exercise duration in response to oral ISDN. Drug was given at 8 am, 1 pm and 6 pm. Exercise tests were performed at 8, 9, 11 am and 1, 2, 4, 6, 7 pm. The duration of exercise was markedly increased after isosorbide. However, the magnitude of this increase progressively declined during the day.

The duration of maximal effect was probably not much greater than 2–3 hours and the magnitude of effect decreased with each succeeding dose during the day. Conventional 3 × daily administration of isosorbide provided major benefit for no more than 6 hours of the 24 hour period. Peak effect was attenuated after the second daily dose and markedly diminished after the third. In commentary, Marcus raises the question as to whether this class of drug is being prescribed appropriately for the majority of patients with stable angina pectoris. He further suggests that a nitroglycerin patch (or isosorbide) should be used with a clear knowledge of the pain pattern in each individual patient. For example post-prandial angina might be treated with either patch or isosorbide in anticipation of an anginal event within 2 hours. Nocturnal angina might be treated with a patch applied at bedtime.

Unstable angina pectoris and the acute coronary syndromes

Little direct information from controlled trials in these conditions is available. Mechanisms are likely to differ because of the role of ulceration and thrombus. Flaherty [10] reported a significant benefit in patients with myocardial infarction receiving nitroglycerin within 10 hours of symptom onset in comparison to placebo. If nitrates act acutely – by whatever mechanism – and such action favorably alters ventricular function, or platelet adhesiveness then the later development of tolerance to continued infusion will not be recognized.

Congestive heart failure

Patients with congestive heart failure are the second large population to receive nitrates, in particular isosorbide dinitrate. Continuous administration of ISDN with hydralazine [6] results in a significant reduction of 20–25% in mortality in patients with Class II–III chronic heart failure, compared to a placebo control and to a group of patients receiving prazosine (a pure vasodilator).

Packer [19] reported on the development of attenuation of the depressor effect of nitroglycerin after 48 hours of continuous intravenous infusion (6.4 micrograms/kilo/min). Intermittent therapy – 12 hours off – did not result in the development of attenuation, or of increase in heart rate or plasma renin activity. In patients who developed tolerance, N-acetylcysteine caused partial reversal of attenuation. DuPuis and colleagues [9] infused nitroglycerin (1.5 micrograms/kilo/min) in 13 patients with congestive heart failure. At 24 hours mean arterial pressure had returned to base line values. The wedge pressure, which had fallen substantively in the first hour also rose towards its control value as did the systemic vascular resistance. Of importance was the clear definition of hemodilution as well as an increase in plasma renin activity. After a 24 hour nitrate free interval values returned towards the preinfusion control. N-acetylcysteine was without effect on the development of tolerance measured by return of mean arterial blood pressure change in pulmonary capillary wedge pressure, pulmonary artery pressure or systemic vascular resistance. However, right arterial pressure remained reduced in patients receiving N-acetylcysteine. These authors concluded that hemodynamic tolerance to nitroglycerin to be multifactorial.

Packer [18] suggests that the development of tolerance to nitroglycerin may be explained by:

1. depletion of sulfhydryl cofactors
2. activation of endogenous vasoconstrictor mechanisms
3. expansion of intravascular volume.

An interesting possibility appears to be that veins rather than arteries may be the primary site of tolerance [24] which is reversible by sulfhydryl cofactors. The expansion of intravascular volume that was not in fact accompanied by an increase in body weight caused by a shift of fluid from the extracellular to the intravascular space. Packer concludes that the available evidence suggests that multiple mechanisms promote the development of tolerance to nitroglycerin in congestive heart failure. The rapid increase in plasma renin activity is consistent with neurohormonal activation and may explain an observation in which nitroglycerin tolerance was modified by an ACE inhibitor. The development of tolerance to nitroglycerin in patients with chronic congestive heart failure appears to be multifactorial and far more complex than heretofore expected.

Current approach to nitrate tolerance

The development of tolerance can be avoided by appropriate dosing intervals to allow the blood and tissue nitrate concentration to approach zero [8]. Nitrate-free intervals of 8 to 12 hours have been recommended – perhaps a median of 10 would be satisfactory. Oral doses must be omitted, transcutaneous patches removed, and, probably, intravenous infusions interrupted. In the latter situation, careful monitoring would be prudent. In patients with chronic stable angina, the clinical history should define those times at which the probability of an ischemic episode is the greatest. A Holter recording might be used to confirm this. Thus in patients in whom activity regulary results in the development of ischemia, would be suitable for an intermittent dosage schedule allowing for a relatively long „unprotected" interval. However, nitrates are not the only drugs useful in the management of myocardial ischemia and chronic stable angina. Beta blockers can be used in association with nitrates and in particular in patients in whom the risk of an acute episode in a nitrate free interval might be relatively great. Its role in unstable angina might well be reevaluated since the fundamental mechanism is not in fact either vasomotion or an increase in oxygen demand, but the presence of thrombus. The value of N-acetylcysteine or ACE inhibitors is at the present time experimental and a definitive answer is not yet available.

In spite of the considerable revival in interest and extensive and imaginative investigative efforts on the basic and clinical level, the actions and uses of nitrates remain complex, with many questions unanswered. Is this due to the general truth: "The more one knows about a phenomenon, the more one realizes the infinity of what one does not know". Or is the issue the specifics of differing biological action and errors in concept resulting from inappropriate extrapolation between different experiments, clinical experiences, and formal clinical trials?

References

[1] Bassan, M. M.: The Antianginal Effect of Long-term 3 Times Daily Administered Isosorbide Dinitrate. JACC. *16* (1990) 936–940.

[2] Bassenge, E., R. Busse: Endothelial modulation of coronary tone. Prog. Cardiovasc. Dis. *30* (1988) 349–380.

[3] Brown, B. G., E. L. Bolson, H. L. Dodge: Dynamic mechanisms in human coronary stenosis. Circ. *70* (1984) 917–922.

[4] Brown, B. G., E. L. Bolson, R. B. Peterson et al.: The mechanism of nitroglycerine action: stenosis vasodilatation as a major component of the drug response. Circ. *64* (1981) 1089–1097.

[5] Chatterjee, K., W. W. Parmley, H. J. C. Swan et al.: Beneficial effects of vasodilators agents in severe mitral regurgitation due to dysfunction of the subvalvar apparatus. Circ. *48* (1973) 684–690.

[6] Cohn, J. N., D. G. Archibald, S. Ziesche et al.: Effect of vasodilator therapy on mortality in chronic congestive heart failure. N. Engl. J. Med. *314* (1986) 1547–1552.

[7] Davies, M. J., A. C. Thomas: Plaque fissuring: The cause of acute myocardial infarction, sudden ischemic death and crescendo angina. Br. Heart J. *53* (1985) 363–373.

[8] DeMonts, H., S. P. Glasser: Intermittent Transdermal Nitroglycerine Therapy in the Treatment of Chronic Stable Angina. JACC. *13* (1989) 786–793.

[9] DuPuis, J., G. Lalonde, R. Lemieux et al.: Tolerance to Intravenous Nitroglycerine in Patients with Congestive Heart Failure: Role of Increased Intravascular Volume, Neurohumoral Activation and Lack of Prevention with N-Acetylcystine JACC. *16* (1990) 923–931.

[10] Flaherty, J. T., P. R. Reid, D. T. Kelly et al.: Intravenous nitroglycerine in acute myocardial infarction. Circ. *51* (1975) 32–37.
[11] Fung, H. L., S. Chong, E. Kowaluk et al.: Mechanisms for the pharmacological interaction of organic nitrates with thiols. Existence of an extracellular pathway for the reversal of nitrate vascular tolerance by N-acetylcysteine. J. Pharm. Exp. Therap. *245* (1988) 524–530.
[12] Furchgott R. F., J. V. Zawadzki: The obligatory role of endothelial cells in the relaxation of arterial smooth muscle by acetylcholine. Nature *288* (1980) 373–376.
[13] Ganz, W., H. S. Marcus: Failure of intracoronary nitroglycerine to alleviate pacing induced angina. Circ. *46* (1972) 880–885.
[14] Ignarro, L. J., H. Lippton, J. C. Edwards et al.: Mechanism of smooth muscle relaxation by organic nitrates, nitrites, nitroprusside, and nitric oxide: evidence for the involvement of S-nitrosothiols as active intermediates. J. Pharmacol. Exp. Ther. *218* (1981) 739–749.
[15] Kelly, R. P., H. Gibbs, M. F. O'Rourke et al.: Nitroglycerine has more favorable effects on the left ventricular afterload than arrant from measurement of pressure in a peripheral artery. Eur. Heart J. *11* (1990) 138–144.
[16] Nabel, E. G., A. P. Selwyn, P. Ganz: Large Coronary Arteries in Humans are Responsive to Changing Blood Flow: An Endothelium Dependent Mechanism That Fails in Patients With Atherosclerosis. JACC. *16* (1990) 349–356.
[17] Needleman, P., E. M. Johnson: Mechanism of tolerance development to organic nitrates. J. Pharmacol. Exp. Ther. *184* (1973) 709–715.
[18] Packer, M.: What Causes Tolerance to Nitroglycerine?: The Hundred year old Mystery Continues. JACC. *16* (1990) 932–935.
[19] Packer, M., W. H. Lee, P. D. Kessler et al.: Prevention and reversal of nitrate tolerence in patients with congestive heart failure. N. Eng. J. Med. *317* (1987) 799–805.
[20] Parker, J. O., B. Farrell, K. A. Lahey et al.: Nitrate Tolerance – the Lack of Effect of N-Acetylcystine. Circ. (1987) 78–572.
[21] Parker, J. O., H. L. Fung, D. Ruggirello et al.: Tolerance to Isosorbide Dinitrate: Rate of Development and Reversal. Circ. 68 (1983) 1074–1080.
[22] Pohl, U., R. Busse: Endothelium-derived relaxing factor inhibits the effects of nitrocompounds in isolated arteries. Am. J. Physiol. 252 (1987) 307–313.
[23] Stewart, D. D.: Remarkable Tolerance to Nitroglycerine. Philadelphia Pollard Clinic 172 (1988).
[24] Stewart, D. J., D. Elsner, O. Sommer et al.: Altered spectrum of nitroglycerine action in long term treatment: nitroglycerine-specific tolerance with mantainance of arterial vasodepressor potency. Civc. *74* (1986) 573–582.
[25] Thadani, U., S. F. Hamilton, E. Olsen et al.: Transdermal Nitroglycerine Patches in Angina Pectoris: Dose Titration, Duration of Effect, and Rapid Tolerance. Ann. Internal Medicine (1986) 105–485.

New pharmacological concepts concerning the active mechanism of organic nitro-compounds

E. Noack

Organic nitro-vasodilators are still the basic therapeutic agents in the treatment of coronary heart disease. In addition, due to their especially pronounced effects on the capacitative resistance vessels in acute pulmonary edema, they are used in the acute reduction of a pathologically increased arterial pressure and in cases of cardiac insufficiency.

Although specific compounds such as volatile amylnitrite or glycerol trinitrate (nitroglycerin) were regularly used therapeutically during the last century, thus belonging to the oldest agents in the medical treasury, little has been known about their exact mechanism of action on a molecular level even up to a few years ago. Two developments have, however, fundamentally changed this. The first resulted in a rapid advance of knowledge due to considerable activity in basic scientific research as it became known that vascular endothelium plays a significant role in the regulation of the local vascular tone and, therewith that radical nitrogen monoxide, NO, in conjunction with vasorelaxing and dilating substances, possibly assumes an important position. Pioneering work in this field was performed in the experiments of Robert Furchgott on isolated vessels. Furchgott and Zawadzky found in 1980, in vascular segments of human A. mammary interna (fig. 1) that concentration-dependant acetylcholine only leads to vasorelaxation as long as intact endothelium is present [6]. The researchers came to the conclusion that the synthesis and release of a substance, set into motion through the influence of acetylcholine in the endothelium, is then able to relax the vascular smooth muscle. This substance was named "Endothelial Derived Relaxing Factor," EDRF, and many more years were then required to definitively clarify the identity of this very short-lived substance.

The second important advance was successfully reached in 1987 when an analytical procedure was found which allowed nitrogen monoxide, NO, to be quantitatively measured in very minimal physiological concentrations. Moncada's research team [2] and my team [2, 3] were both successful in this respect, in close succession, through the utilization of very different analytic methods. While the Moncada team proved chemiluminescence as a sensitive, but also

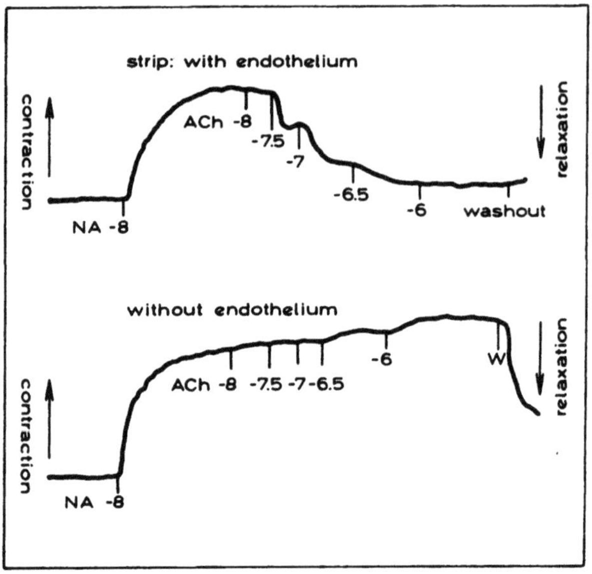

Fig. 1 Isolated vascular strips of a rat aorta were precontracted with 10 nM of noradrenaline before (upper part) and after (lower part) mechanical removal of the epithelial layer.
The subsequent application of increasing concentration of acetylcholine (10 nM to 1 μM) resulted in a differing vasorelaxatory behaviour (modified according to lit. [6]).

technically expensive method, we adapted a spectrophotometric process, which made use of the NO-dependant transformation of oxyhemoglobin to methemoglobin. The latter method had, above all, the advantage of high specificity, and it was thereby possible to carry out continuous measurements for the first time. In this manner we were successful in confirming the long assumed hypothesis, with various technical methods, that the EDRF released by vascular endothelium is identical with nitrogen monoxide (NO).

NO is a colorless gas with a high lipid solubility. This makes it possible for the compound to rapidly penetrate the blood stream, after luminal endothelium diffusion and the vascular wall into the smooth muscle cells, after abluminal diffusion. The next figure (fig. 2) shows the molecule in which the nitrogen and oxygen atoms are closely connected spatially with each other. NO possesses an uneven number of electrons, which makes it especially reactive. It quickly

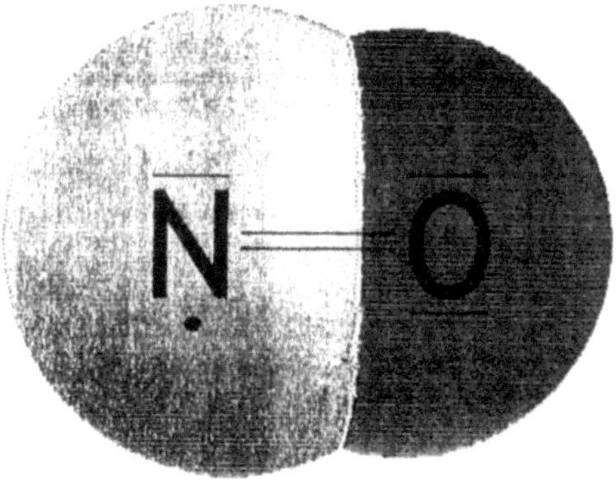

Fig. 2 Chemical structure of radical nitrogen monoxide, NO. Note the uneven number of 11 electrons causing the high reactivity of the compound.

decomposes, within a few seconds, in solutions containing oxygen forming nitrite and nitrate anions. In nanomolar concentrations it has a particularly relaxing effect on arterial vessels, and prevents thrombocyte adhesion and aggregation.

Although the organic compounds differ greatly in their chemical structure, they both possess an oxidized nitrogen portion. This is the point of departure for differing bioactivation reactions whose end result are, uniformly, the formation of radical NO. Of course, the rates with which the individual organic nitro compounds such as ISDN, nitroglycerin, or molsidomine form NO are very different. Investigations of the last few years clearly substantiate that NO is the true activator of the key enzyme responsible for relaxation in smooth muscle cells: the cytosolic soluble guanylate cyclase. It is thereby the initiator for relaxation and decrease in tone in the vessels (fig. 3). Activation of guanylate cyclase results in the increased formation of cyclic GMP from guanosine triphosphate, GTP. The number of cGMP produced corresponds directly with the concentration of NO available. Also when NO is temporarily stored in reactive intermediary compounds, like the so-called nitrosothiols, which under in vivo conditions is quite possible, the final enzyme activation is always dependant on the NO molecule itself. This is also supported by our in vitro experiments with isolated guanylate cyclase [2]. If we were to choose experimental conditions under which all tested nitrovasodilators are half-maximally activated by the

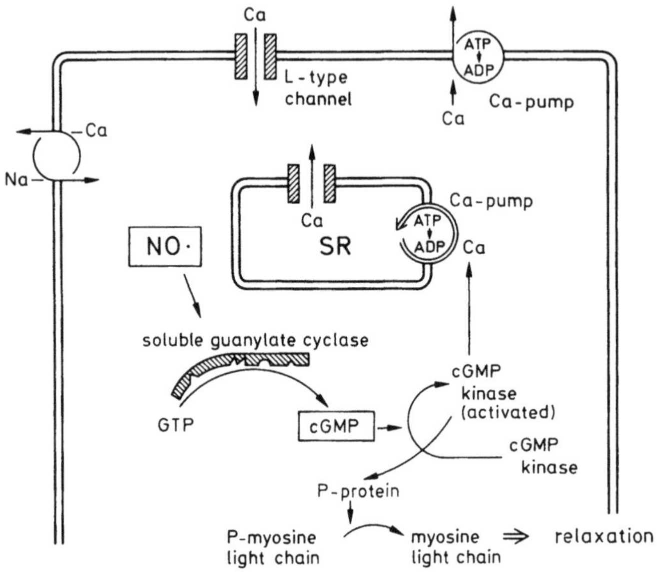

Fig. 3 Schematic presentation of a vascular smooth muscle cell explaining the molecular mechanism with which NO, through the activation of the soluble guanylate cyclase reduces the cellular calcium concentration producing a reduction of vascular tone. See text for further details.

Organic nitrate	EC_{50} (mM)	NO-release μM/min
GTN	0.069	0.050
IMDN	0.200	0.045
IIDN	0.242	0.047
ISDN	0.280	0.046
IS-2-N	0.750	0.047
IS-5-N	1.050	0.045

Fig. 4 Concentrations of organic nitrates which lead to the halfmaximal activation of soluble guanylate cyclase always release the same amounts of NO per time unit. GTN = glycerol trinitrate, IMDN = Isomannide-dinitrate, IIDN = Isoidide-dinitrate, ISDN = Isosorbide-dinitrate, IS-2-N = Isosorbide-2-mononitrate, IS-5-N = Isosorbide-5-mononitrate.

enzyme gualylate cyclase, we could then show with our direct NO measurement method, that the velocity of released NO is identical (fig. 4), and, therefore, behaves independently of the chemical constitution of the compound containing NO.

Under in vivo conditions, the cGMP formed, as a kind of second messenger, accelerates a series of phosphorylation processes in the smooth vascular muscle cells, which ultimately result in the relaxation of the vessels. It is unclear by which molecular mechanism cGMP decreases the cytosolic Ca^{2+} concentration and leads to relaxation. One of the partial reactions could concern the quick restorage of intracellularly released calcium in the sarcoplasmic reticulum. It is known that phospholambane is a cellular regulator protein through which cyclic nucleotide is phosphorylated. This also occurs in the vascular muscle cells. Karczewski et al [7] recently demonstrated that NO (100 μM) and ATP (50 μM) lead to an increase in phosphorylation of phospholambane in the intact vascular wall in isolated segments of the rat aorta, parallel to that of the measured vascular relaxation. The stimulation of the re-uptake reaction for Ca^{2+} by NO could reflect the discovery of a decisive mechanism for the vessel-dilatating effect of EDRF and NO, and thereby the organic nitrovasodilators. This could also explain why organic nitro-compounds distinctly improve compliance of the vessel walls of large arteries.

As previously indicated, NO is principally released from therapeutically applied organic nitro-compounds with differing velocities. Different biochemical and chemical mechanisms have a regulatory function in the required bioactivation processes. The primary reaction is dependant on the chemical nature of the drug. Thus, for example, the classic organic nitrates such as nitroglycerin are metabolized to NO by two different mechanisms: an enzymatic and a non-enzymatic bioactivation pathway.

In principle, the compound must first succeed in entering the smooth muscle cells in intact form before it is bioactivated to NO because the effect of NO is restricted to small distances, due to its high chemical instability and its particular reactivity. Our investigations of structure-activity relationships in isolated, perfused Langendorff hearts [12], have shown that the extent of the vessel-relaxing effect directly corresponds to the lipophilicity of the individual organic nitrate (fig. 5). This provides a realistic explanation for the much greater efficacy of glycerol trinitate, on a molar basis, over isosorbide dinitrate (ISDN) and for that of ISDN over, in turn, isosorbide-5-mononitrate. Therefore, the mere increase in fat-solubility of a nitrate will correspondingly increase its efficacy.

The steric configuration, i. e. the sterical structure, of the nitrate group in the endo- and exo-position has an additional modulating effect in ring-containing

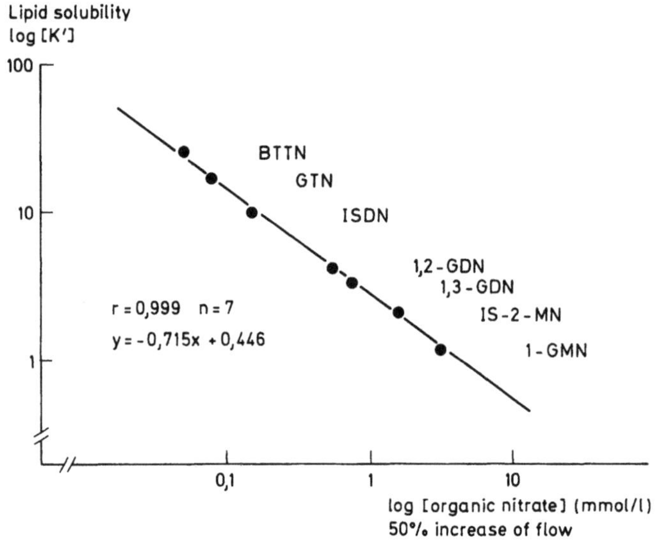

Fig. 5 Double logarithmic plot of the relationship between lipophililicity and the concentrations of organic nitro-compounds, which increase the coronary flow in isolated guinea pig hearts by 50%.
BTTN = 1,2,4-butantriol-trinitrate, 1,2-GDN = 1,2-glycerine dinitrate,
1-GMN = 1-glycerine mononitrate (compare also fig. 4).

nitrocompounds. The penetration of compounds containing an exo-positioned nitro-group is favoured, due to the more elongated shape, producing less sterical hindrance when entering the cell membrane. At the same time, the compound is pharmacologically more effective than the isomer with an endo-positioned nitro group. This holds true for both mononitrates of isosorbide as well as for teopranitol, a symbiontic substance (fig. 6), representing an isosorbide-5-mononitrate linked in the 2-position with a theophylline derivative yielding four stereoisomers (2-exo/5-exo = KC 046; 2-endo/5-exo = K 116; 2-exo/5-endo = KC 144 and 2-endo/5-endo = KC 146). Our results, reproduced in fig. 7, confirm the expected varying relaxing effect on the coronary vessel tone in isolated perfused Langendorff hearts by the four teopranitol isomers (fig. 7). As may be seen, the two isomers with an exo-positioned nitrate group in the 5-position cause the significantly strongest vascular relaxation (2-endo/5-exo and 2-exo/5-endo). In contrast all four examined stereo isomers differ only slightly from one another in the rate of NO release and thus in the degree of enzyme activation.

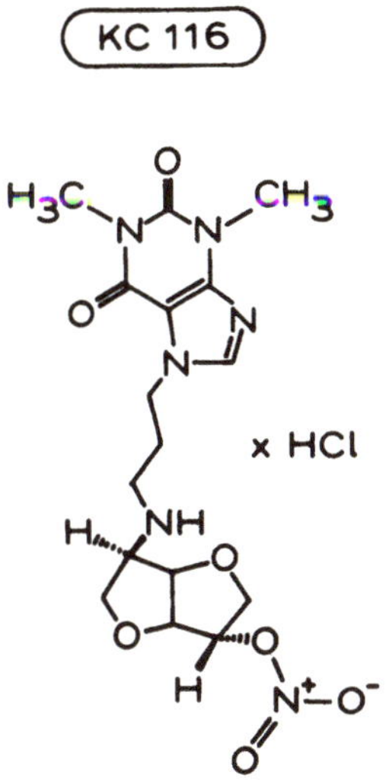

Fig. 6 Structural formula of teopranitol (KC 116).

Concerning the bioactivation of organic nitrates, enzymatic and purely chemical degradation pathways are able to compete with each other in the smooth muscle cells. Enzymatic break-down processes are especially significant when the concentrations of the active ingredient are minimal. The most extensively examined process in this respect is the catalytic biotransformation through glutathione-S-transferase. Most of the resulting final products are nitrite anions. Our experimental results confirm that a stimulation of the guanylate cyclase is quite uncertain because NO is only produced in minimal concentrations. As far as the organic nitrate degradation of biologically active substances is concerned, this reaction represents a dead end resulting in a waste of vasoactive substances. Recently, other enzymatic metabolic pathways have been found which may be of pharmacological significance. Servent et al. [20] recently described the formation of a complex compound of NO and cytochrome when glycerol trinitrate was incubated with rat liver microsomes. The formation preceded a NADPH-dependant denitrification. To what extent this type of enzyme-system also occurs in the smooth vascular muscle cells must, however, first be clarified.

On the other hand, organic nitrates are already bioactivated in vitro if specific thiol-containing compounds, such as cystein or acetylcystein are present. In addition to NO, nitrite anions in a ratio of approximately 1:14 and, in very small amounts, nitrate anions also appear (fig. 8). The more alkaline the envi-

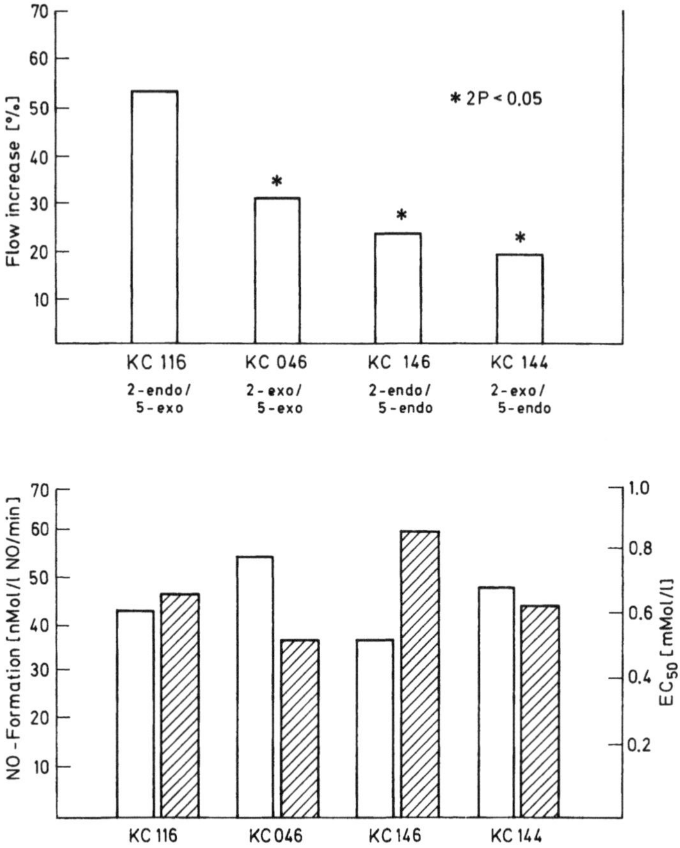

Fig. 7 Percent increase of the coronary flow by four stereo-isomeric forms of teopranitol in isolated perfused guinea pig hearts according to Langendorff (above section of figure). Relationship between the NO-release from the four teopranitol stereoisomers and the half-maximal activation of soluble guanylate cyclase (EC_{50} values).

ronment, the more quickly the reaction proceeds, as free thiolate anions, apparently essential to the initiation of the bioactivation process, form from undissociated thiols as the pH rises. Apparently a reactive intermediate compound is formed from the interaction of cystein and organic nitrate, from which biologically active NO and biologically inert nitrite are produced as reaction products. During the reaction, the nucleophilic thiolate anion is able to react with the

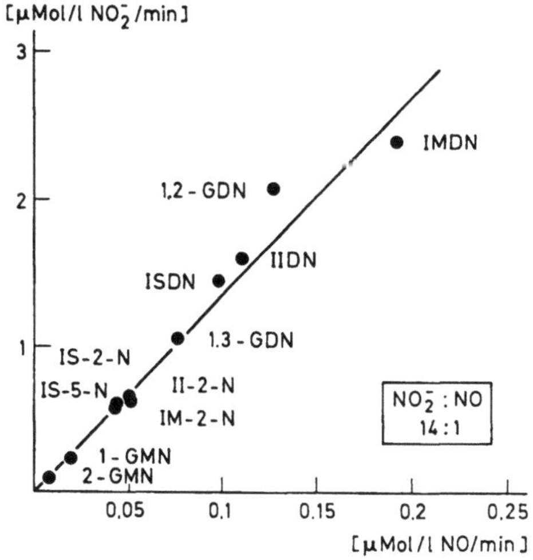

Fig. 8 Correlation between NO- and nitrite-formation from organic nitrates in vitro in the presence of 5 mM of cystein. (Abbr. see figs. 4 and 5).

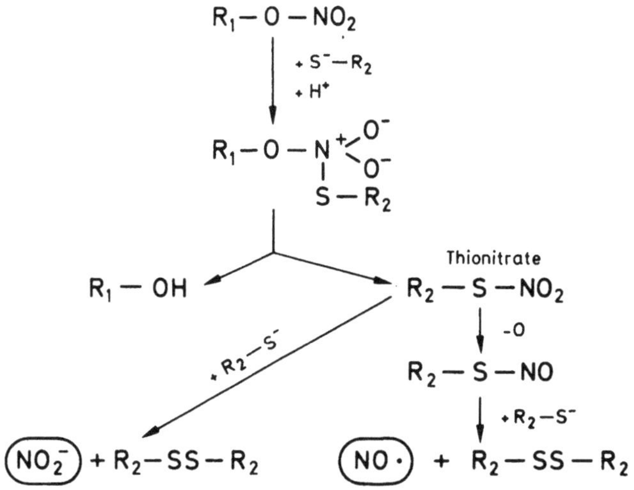

Fig. 9 Molecular processes which lead to the formation of NO and nitrite from organic nitrates. See text for details.

nitrogen atom of the organic nitrate in such a way that a thiolate ester is produced through trans-esterisation (fig. 9). Finally, a thio-ester, highly unstable in an aqueous solution, might quickly degrade to NO and nitrite after reduction. It is possible that part of the resulting NO thereby becomes temporarily stabilized by cystein in the form of a nitrosothiol.

In this respect it is interesting that NO has a high affinity to various metal complexes, such as the iron-containing hem-group of oxy-hemoglobin or of guanylate cyclase. A Russian research team was able to show that glycerol trinitrate in vivo is broken down by the release of radical NO, which then reacts, with iron and hemoglobin-containing proteins, forming nitrosyl-protein complexes [8]. A comparable reaction could take place between organic nitrates and the guanylate cyclase itself. In this case, the enzyme itself would overtake an active role in the metabolism or bioactivation of the various nitrovasodilators. In fact, many cystein molecules are found in the environment of the active center of guanylate cyclase, i. e. in the heme-portion, which thus may possess a similar bioactivatory function to that which I described above for the degredation of the compounds in an aqueous solution in the presence of cystein. The guanylate cyclase, therefore, would then be at least theoretically in a position to actively take part in the bioactivation mechanism of the organic nitrates.

As both the enzymatic and non-enzymatic degradation of organic nitrates are essentially dependant on the availability of special thiol compounds, it is easily explained that the exhaustion, particularly of the cystein pool, results in a slower bioactivation process, as has been shown in many investigations. The clinical correlation of these intracellular changes is the so-called nitrate tolerance, which can only be avoided through the strict observance of certain therapy guidelines. Remarkably, amylnitrite, nitrosothiol and sodium nitroprusside also release NO in noteworthy amounts even if cystein is not present, and nevertheless, do not show any signs of tolerance in isolated vessels [15]. This strongly supports the possibility that changes in the thiol content of smooth muscle cells favor or are the essential cause of a nitrate tolerance [13].

It is interesting to notice that small coronary resistance vessels with a diameter of $< 100\ \mu m$, in contrast to larger coronary arteries, do not respond to the application of nitroglycerin by vasodilatation. Selke et al. (1990) recently showed that this could be due to the fact that the small vessels have no facilities to transform nitroglycerin into its active species [18]. It is possible that the necessary reservoir of SH-containing compounds necessary for bioactivation is not available in this vessel-type. This hypothesis is indirectly supported by Kurz [9] in trials on dog hearts in situ, in which exogenously added L-cystein (100 μM) brought about a relaxation of the coronary arteries with a diameter below 100 μM in the presence of 10 μM of nitroglycerin. The activity of guanylate cyclase in human platelets is also only stimulated by nitroglycerin in the presence of cystein [16]. All these findings support our in vitro data, according to which the bioactivation of organic nitrates, like that of nitroglycerin, demands the interaction with specific SH-containing compounds, preferably cystein.

The new chemical class of furoxanes, which was discovered as a consequence of the continuous activities in sydnonimine chemistry, possesses a distinctly different bioactivation pathway. They are NO-containing compounds which cause a strong vasodilatory effect in isolated perfused hearts and in intact animal trials. While the release of NO from some compounds is completely independent of the presence of thiol-containing substances, the activity of others is more quickly accelerated by a factor of 10 or higher. Fig. 10 shows, for example, the different behavior of 3 typical furoxane derivatives. It is important to notice, in this context, that the type of thiol-containing compound present is completely unimportant. In contrast to classical organic nitrates, only the presence of the SH-group is essential for the initiation of the bioactivation steps. As thiols are ubiquitous in the organism, the tendency of a tolerance development is only minimal or not existent at all.

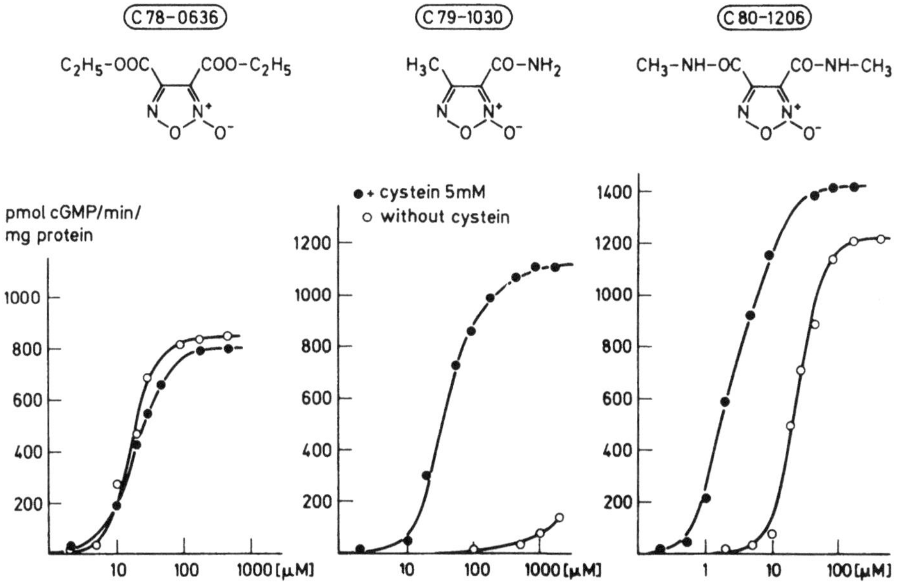

Fig. 10 Activation of crude, soluble guanylate cyclase by various furoxane derivatives in the presence and absence of 5 mM of cystein.

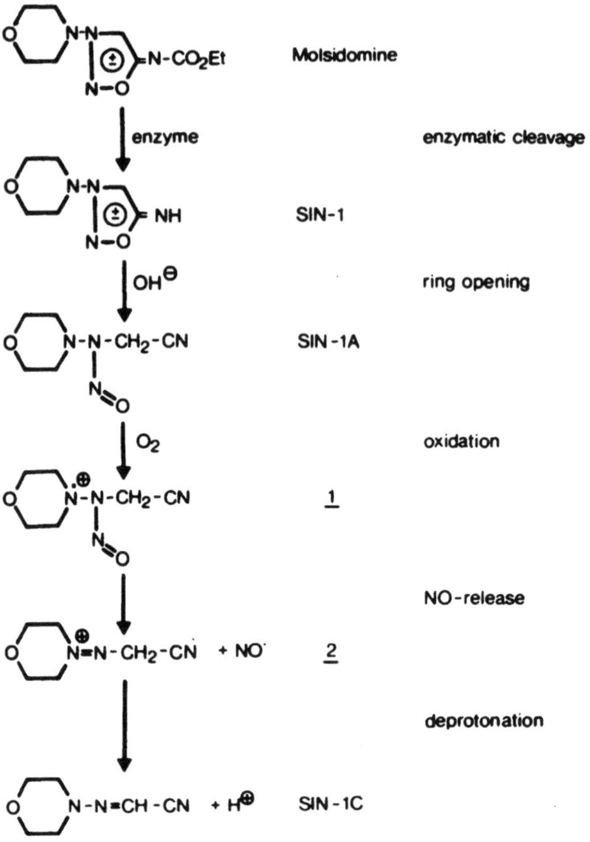

Fig. 11 Bioactivation pathway of molsidomine, which leads to the release of radical NO representing the pharmacological, active compound.

This applies also to the sydnonimines, of which molsidomine is the best-known and therapeutically used. During the last 2 years the most important steps in the complicated bioactivation pathway of this chemical class have been elucidated [1, 4, 14]. The next figure (fig. 11) shows the biotransformation pathway in which the NO-release from the open-ring SIN-1A-derivative is the critical step for the development of the pharmacological effect. As we know only recently, the presence of small amounts of oxygen is an absolute prerequisite. As other oxidants also accelerate the bioactivation process, it is obvious that an oxidative process is required for the breakdown of SIN-1A (fig. 11), which is initiated by

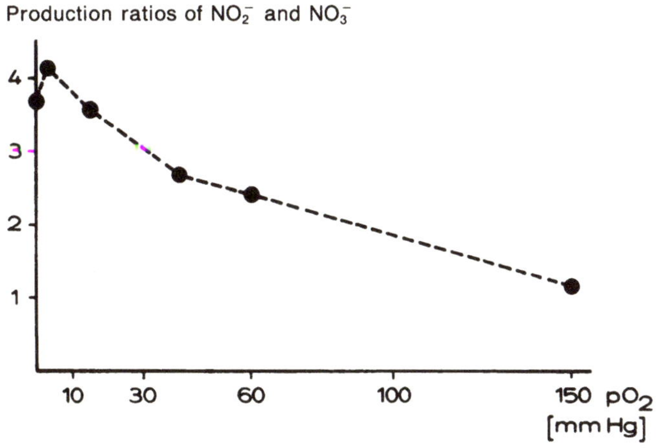

Fig. 12 Influence of oxygen tension on the velocity of formation of nitrite and nitrate anions from SIN-1, the primary metabolite of molsidomine. Even small amounts of oxygen are sufficient to guarantee a substantial formation of nitrite.

the oxidation of the nitrogen atom belonging to the morpholine ring. At the same time, an electron passes to the oxygen molecule, forming O_2^-. Of course, a few oxygen molecules are sufficient for the ultimate liberation of NO, so that a therapeutically sufficient amount of NO in vivo can be guaranteed in ischemic tissue areas. On the other hand, our experiments show that the formation of other pharmacologically inactive reaction-products, like those from organic nitrite and nitrate are, in part, strongly influenced by the oxygen content of the surrounding environment (fig. 12).

In summary, our results show that all therapeutically applied nitrovasodilators represent prodrugs from which, in very different ways, an intracellular release of NO for the activation of guanylate cyclase takes place. As was shown in the case of sydnonimines, oxidative pathways are involved which resemble the physiological, enzyme-mediated formation of NO from L-arginine [11]. The final biologically active compound is always nitrogen monoxide, NO, while the formation of an organic nitrite or nitrate is either due to secondary reactions, like the oxidation of NO, or by parallel reactions. They are biologically inactive end products even though they occur in relatively high concentrations. We believe that the particular dependency of the bioactivation of organic nitrate on the presence of special thiol-containing compounds is the explanation for the pronounced tendency during prolonged application to develop nitrate tolerance.

The long-term, known nitrovasodilators, which were generally discovered by chance, still do not represent the ideal therapeutical solution. However, now that there is a better understanding of the molecular processes in bioactivation, the opportunity to develop novel compounds which orient themselves more towards the physiological pathways of NO-generation would surely be worthwhile. Arginine- or nitrato-cystein derivates would be, for example, conceivable alternatives [22]. Furthermore, the organic nitrates appear in a totally new light clinically, especially concerning their possible role in the treatment of ischemic tissue damage [16]. NO has a remarkable affinity to oxygen radicals with which it quickly reacts forming peroxynitrites which, in turn, separate into molecular oxygen and nitrate ions. Thus nitrovasodilators could exert, in addition to their indirect relieving effect on the heart and their direct NO substituting activity, a direct protective effect in ischemia and reperfusion. Thus, the considerable efforts in basic research in the last years have renewed the therapeutical interest in nitrovasodilators, which due to their comprehensive pharmacological activity may introduce a new era in the treatment of ischemic heart disease, especially if new NO-liberating drugs are launched into therapy.

The experimental work was supported by the Deutsche Forschungsgemeinschaft (SFB 242 Düsseldorf, Coronary Heart Disease, Teilprojekt C 3 NOACK).

References

[1] Bohn, H., K. Schönafinger: Oxygen and oxidation promote the release of nitric oxide from sydnonimines. J. Cardiovasc. Pharmacol. *14* (Suppl. 11) (1989) 6–12.

[2] Feelisch, M., E. Noack: Correlation between nitric oxide formation during degeneration of organic nitrates and activation of guanylate cyclase. Eur. J. Pharmacol. *139* (1987) 19–30.

[3] Feelisch, M., E. Noack: Nitric oxide (NO) formation from nitrovasodilators occurs independently of hemoglobin or non-heme iron. Eur. J. Pharmacol. *142* (1987) 465–469.

[4] Feelisch, M., E. Noack: On the mechanism of NO release from sydnonimines. J. Cardiovasc. Pharmacol. *14* (Suppl. 11) (1989) 13–22.

[5] Feelisch, M., E. Noack: The in vitro metabolism of nitrovasodilators and their conversion into vasoactive species. In: B. S. Lewis, A. Kimichi (Hrsg.): Heart failure – mechanisms and management, pp. 241–255. Springer-Verlag Berlin, Heidelberg 1991.

[6] Furchgott, R. F., J. V. Zawadzki: The obligatory role of endothelial cells in the relaxation of arterial smooth muscle by acetylcholine. Nature *288* (1980) 373–376.

[7] Karczewski, P., M. Kelm, M. Hartmann et al.: Bedeutung von Phospholamban bei der Endothel-vermittelten Relaxation der Rattenaorta. Z. Kardiol. *79* (Suppl. 1) (1990) Abstr. 212, 64.

[8] Kuropteva, Z. V., O. N. Pastuschenko: Change in paramagnetic blood and liver complexes in animals under the influence of nitroglycerin. Dokl. Akad. Nauk. SSSR *281* (1) (1985) 189–192.
[9] Kurz, M. A.: Mechanisms responsible for the heterogeneous coronary microvascular response to nitroglycerin. Circulation *82* (Suppl. III) (1990) III–N.
[10] Marletta, M. A., P. S. Yoon, R. Iyengar et al.: Macrophage oxidation of L-arginine to nitrite and nitrate: nitric oxide is an intermediate. Biochemistry *27* (1988) 8706–8711.
[11] Noack, E.: Investigation on structure-activity relationship in organic nitrates. Meth. and Find. Exptl. Clin. Pharmacol. *6* (1984) 583–586.
[12] Noack, E.: Mechanism of nitrate tolerance – influence of the metabolic activation pathway. Z. Kardiol. *79* (Suppl. 3) (1990) 51–55.
[13] Noack, E., M. Feelisch: Molecular aspects underlying the vasodilator action of molsidomine. J. Cardiovasc. Pharmacol. *14* (Suppl. 11) (1989) 1–5.
[14] Noack, E. und M. Feelisch: Molecular mechanisms of nitrovasodilator bioactivation. In: H. Drexler et al. (Eds.): Endothelial mechanisms of vasomotor control, pp. 37–50. Steinkopff Verlag, Darmstadt 1991.
[15] Noack, E., M. Murphy: Vasodilation and oxygen radical scavenging by nitric oxide/EDRF and organic nitrovasodilators. In: H. Sies (Hrsg.): „Oxidative Stress II", Academic Press Limited (1991).
[16] Noack, E., H. Schröder, M. Feelisch: Continuous determination of nitric oxide formation during non-enzymatic degradation of organic nitrates and its correlation to guanylate cyclase activation. Naunyn Schmiedeberg's Arch. Pharmacol. (Suppl.) (1986) 125.
[17] Schöttler, B.: Untersuchungen zum molekularen Wirkungsmechanismus der organischen Nitrate an Thrombozyten. Dissertation, Heinrich-Heine-Universität Düsseldorf (1991).
[18] Selke, F. W., R. J. Tomanek, D. G. Harrison: L-Cysteine selectively potentiates dilation of small coronary arterioles by nitroglycerin. Circulation *82* (Suppl. III) (1990) Abstr. 2792 III–703.
[19] Servent, D, M. Delaforge, C. Ducrocq et al.: Nitric oxide formation during microsomal hepatic denitration of glyceryl trinitrate: involvement of cytochrom P–450. Biochem. Biophys. Res. Commun. *163* (1989) 1210–1216.
[20] Palmer, R. M. J., A. G. Ferrige, S. Moncada: Nitric oxide release accounts for the biological activity of endothelium-derived relaxing factor. Nature *327* (1987) 524–526.
[21] Thomas, G., M. Farhat, A. K. Myers et al.: Effect of Nα-benzoyl-L-arginine ethyl ester on coronary perfusion pressure in isolated guinea pig heart. Eur. J. Pharmacol. *178* (1990) 251–254.

Nitroglycerin offsets age-related increase of left ventricular afterload in man – a hidden mechanism exposed

M. O'Rourke, A. Avolio, R. Kelly

Nitroglycerin is an extraordinary effective drug for treatment of angina pectoris and of left ventricular failure [19, 31, 33, 35]. Reasons for such efficacy have been extensively debated in the past (as in a special recent supplement of the European Heart Journal [9]). In the absence of any consistent decrease of peripheral resistance with therapeutic doses, beneficial actions have been attributed to venodilation [31, 33, 35, 9], and in patients with angina pectoris, to dilation of coronary arteries, collateral vessels and eccentric stenoses [4].

Work conducted in Sydney has established that nitroglycerin causes substantial reduction of left ventricular afterload in mature adult humans [12], and probably as a consequence of subtle changes in the calibre and distensibility of small conduit arteries. This effect (fig. 1) is not apparent when blood pressure is recorded conventionally either directly or indirectly from the brachial or radial artery, and is attributable to reduction in pulse wave reflection.

This paper reviews briefly the research that has led up to these findings. While the definitive papers have been published only during 1989 and 1990, they are based on research initiated in 1963 to determine the implications of pulsatility of blood flow to arterial pressure and to cardiac load and function.

The first step (taken in 1963) was to establish the relationship between pulsatile and steady components of arterial pressure and flow as vascular impedance in experimental animals. Data were taken from peripheral and central arteries [22, 29, 30] both under control conditions and during infusion of vasoactive drugs. This work was based on the earlier theoretical and experimental studies of Womersley [44, 45], McDonald [17] and Taylor [37, 38] in the 1950s, and established the important role of wave reflection in determining pulsatile pressure/flow relationships, the contour of arterial pressure and flow waves, and the hydraulic load presented to the left ventricle by the whole systemic circulation. Effects of vasoactive agents could be attributed to change in the intensity and timing of wave reflection [22, 29, 30]. Explanations were aided by modelling

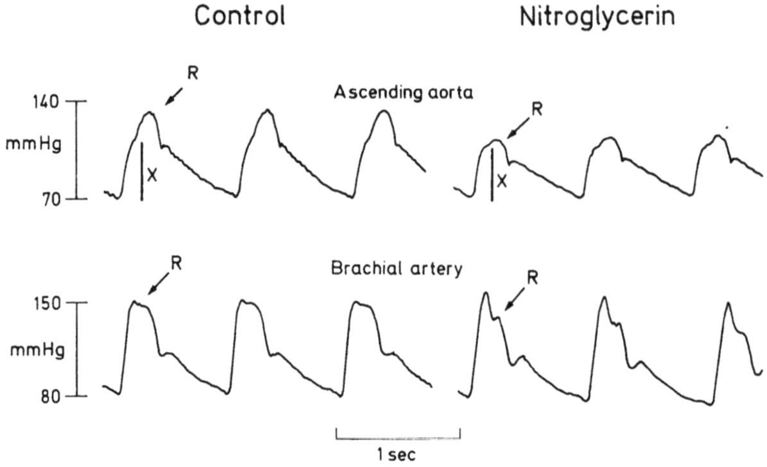

Fig. 1 Pressure waves recorded by a catheter-tip manometer in the ascending aorta (top) and brachial artery (bottom) of a patient with coronary atherosclerosis before (left) and five minutes after (right) administration of 0.3 mg nitroglycerin sublingually. In this patient, aortic systolic pressure decreased by almost 20 mm Hg whereas there was no reduction in brachial systolic pressure. Reduction in aortic systolic pressure was mainly caused by a decrease in the late systolic wave (R); there was little change in amplitude of the initial systolic wave (X). From Kelly et al. [12].

studies conducted concurrently by Michael Taylor, in whose department the experiments were conducted [39, 40]. Taylor and McDonald [18] showed that wave reflection is an inevitable consequence of vascular design, and results from low resistance conduit arteries terminating in high resistance arterioles. Taylor explained how wave reflection under normal circumstances in experimental animals is so timed as to aid cardiac function. This is achieved through a type of "tuning" between the heart and vascular tree [39, 41].

When similar human data were obtained in the late 1960s and 1970s, these concepts did not appear to apply [20, 21, 27]. The same evidence of "tuning" was not in evidence. In most human subjects from whom data were obtained, wave reflection appeared to hinder rather than aid cardiac function. The systolic arterial system in mature adult appeared to be "detuned" from the heart, with wave reflection returning early, boosting systolic pressure in the ascending aorta and left ventricle (rather than pressure in early diastole), [23, 24, 26] (fig. 2). The reasons for this situation became more apparent when attention was directed at

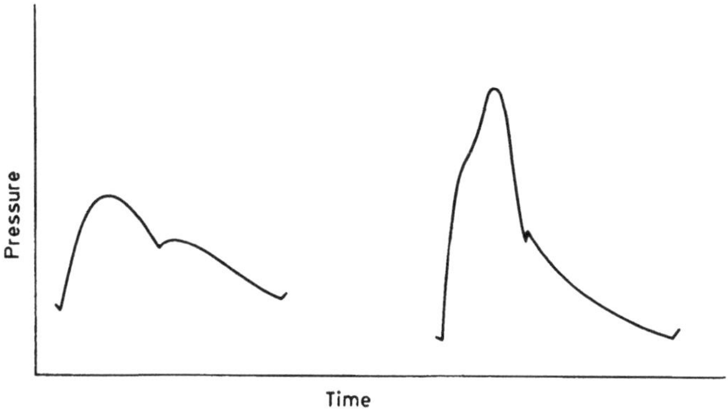

Fig. 2 Typical ascending aortic pressure waves in a young human adult (left) and in a middle aged subject (right). The principal difference is attributable to early wave reflection in the older subject. The reflected wave provides a diastolic undulation in the younger subject. In the older subject the wave returns earlier and causes augmentation of the systolic pressure peak; pressure during diastole falls almost exponentially.

the change in arterial pulse wave velocity with age. By age 50, aortic pulse wave velocity in man is almost twice that in childhood and almost twice that recorded in experimental animals [1] (fig. 3). Increase in aortic wave velocity with age was attributed to arterial stiffening, and established as an aging change, accelerated by hypertension and largely independent of concomitant atherosclerosis [1, 2]. These findings supported the much earlier and largely forgotten impressions of Roy [32] and of Bramwell and Hill [3] who had stressed the importance of progressive arterial stiffening with age in man as an impediment to efficient cardiac function.

With wave reflection in man seen as an impediment rather than an aid to left ventricular function, Yaginuma et al. [42] in Sydney set out to see how this could be modified to the heart's advantage. They showed that nitroglycerin does indeed reduce wave reflection, even though the drug does not decrease peripheral resistance. The effect was to cause a substantial (19 mm Hg) decrease in ascending aortic and left ventricular systolic pressure but no change in aortic diastolic pressure; the small fall in mean pressure (9 mm Hg) was attributed to reduction in venous return and consequently in stroke volume. Modelling studies [26] were utilised to explain experimental findings and an explanation was advanced on the basis of data previously published by Simon et al. [34], Fichett [6], Westling [43], and Feldman et al. [5]. These collectively, indicated that nitroglycerin has

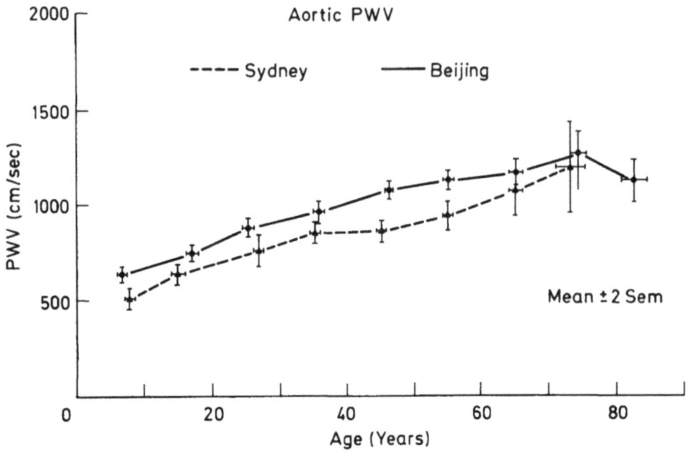

Fig. 3 Changes in pulse wave velocity with age in human subjects from Sydney and Beijing. After Avolio et al. [1].

very potent vasodilatory effects on the smallest conduit arteries while having little or no effect on calibre of the largest conduit arteries (such as the aorta) or on the arterioles. Reduction in wave reflection with nitroglycerin was attributable to relatively greater dilation of daughter branches compared to the parent vessel at an arterial bifurcation (fig. 4). Subsequently, these findings were confirmed by Fitchett et al. [8] and by Latson et al. [16], who concurred with the interpretation given by the Sydney group. Subsequently too, Takazawa [36] with Yaginuma et al. [42] confirmed findings in Japanese subjects.

Significance of these findings was initially overlooked. It was assumed that any reduction in aortic and left ventricular pressure would also be apparent in brachial and radial artery pressure. Since systolic pressure in these arteries usually changed little with normal therapeutic doses of nitroglycerin, it was considered that the large reductions demonstrated by Yaginuma et al. [42], Simkus et al. [7] and Takazawa [36] were a consequence of other factors operating in patients undergoing cardiac catheterisation.

This assumption (of similar reduction in central and peripheral systolic pressure with nitroglycerin) was questioned when we began to utilise a new applanation tonometer, developed jointly in association with Huntley Millar and Dean Winter from Texas [14, 15]. In Sydney we were able to establish that the carotid pressure wave recorded with the tonometer is similar to the ascending aortic pressure wave [15], while the radial pressure wave is quite different, but similar to that

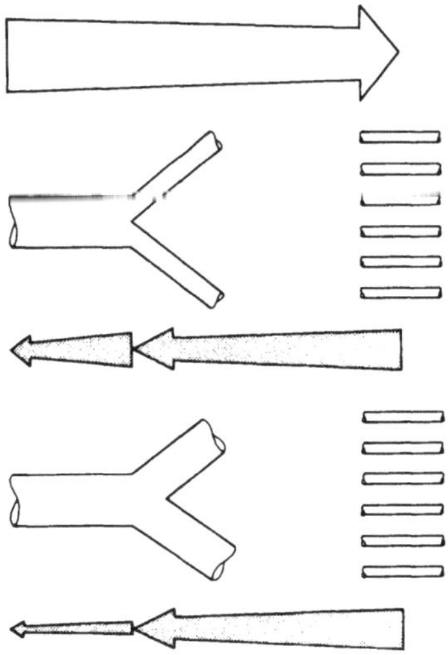

Fig. 4 Proposed mechanism for reduction in wave reflection with nitroglycerin. A wave travelling from the heart (white arrow, above) is reflected at the peripheral arterioles (narrow tubes at right). Under normal circumstances, the reflected wave (grey arrow, centre) is not altered at bifurcations in the arterial tree, whereas during nitroglycerin therapy, the reflected wave (grey arrow, below) is reduced in amplitude as a result of increased dilation of daughter branches at arterial bifurcations. From Yaginuma et al. [42].

recorded invasively in the radial (or brachial) artery [14]. With nitroglycerin, there is far greater reduction in the systolic peak of the carotid pressure wave than in the peak of the radial pressure wave (which often does not decrease at all) [36], (fig. 5). The contour of both waves undergoes a change with nitroglycerin. In the carotid artery there is a late systolic peak, attributable to wave reflection, whereas in the radial artery there is no such peak during late systole. Loss of the late systolic pressure peak in the carotid artery is always accompanied by decrease in amplitude of the late systolic shoulder in the radial artery (fig. 5). However since this does not constitute the peak of the pulse, systolic pressure does not appear to fall (fig. 5). These findings suggested firstly that wave reflection in man has different effects on the contour of the pressure pulse in the ascending aorta and central arteries compared to the countour of the pulse in the radial and brachial arteries, and secondly that measurements of systolic pressure in the brachial or radial arteries may underestimate the reduction in systolic pressure caused by nitroglycerin in the ascending aorta.

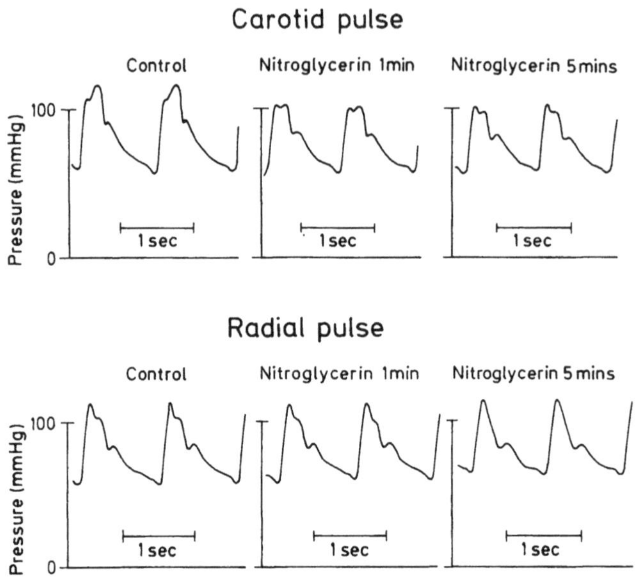

Fig. 5 Pressure waves recorded noninvasively by applanation tonometry in the carotid artery (above) and radial artery (below) of a 50 year old man under control conditions (left), then one minute (centre) and five minutes (right) after administration of nitroglycerin 0.3 mg sublingually. From O'Rourke [28].

The first of these points was confirmed by us [13] in a study of over 1000 normal subjects. This showed progressive changes in contour and amplitude of the central and peripheral pressure pulse with age (fig. 6). Early wave reflection appeared to cause augmentation of systolic pressure in the carotid artery from the fourth decade of life, whereas such augmentation was not apparent in the radial artery until after the eighth decade. In middle aged man wave reflection was responsible for augmentation of systolic pressure in the carotid artery but not in the radial artery. Other data indicated that wave reflection caused a greater degree of systolic pressure augmentation in the ascending aorta than in the carotid artery [13, 15]. What we were able to measure non-invasively in the carotid artery underestimated the boost in systolic pressure provided by wave reflection in the ascending aorta and left ventricle.

The differential effect of nitroglycerin on central and peripheral systolic pressure was confirmed in an invasive study performed prior to cardiac catheterisation in 14 patients with coronary disease prior to coronary angiography [12]. In these

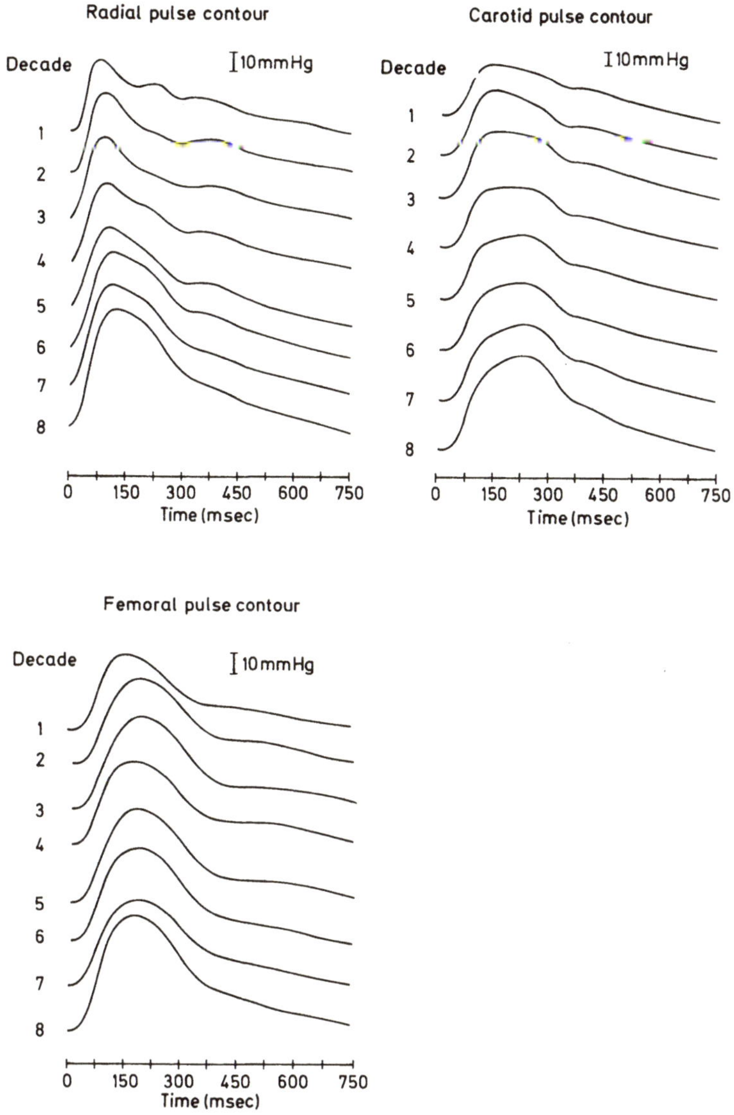

Fig. 6 Change in pressure wave contour, recorded by applanation tonometry, with age in the radial artery (left), carotid artery (right) and femoral artery (below). Each wave represents the ensemble-averaged waves from 40–70 subjects within an age decade group. Data are shown for the first to eighth decade of life. From Kelly et al. [13].

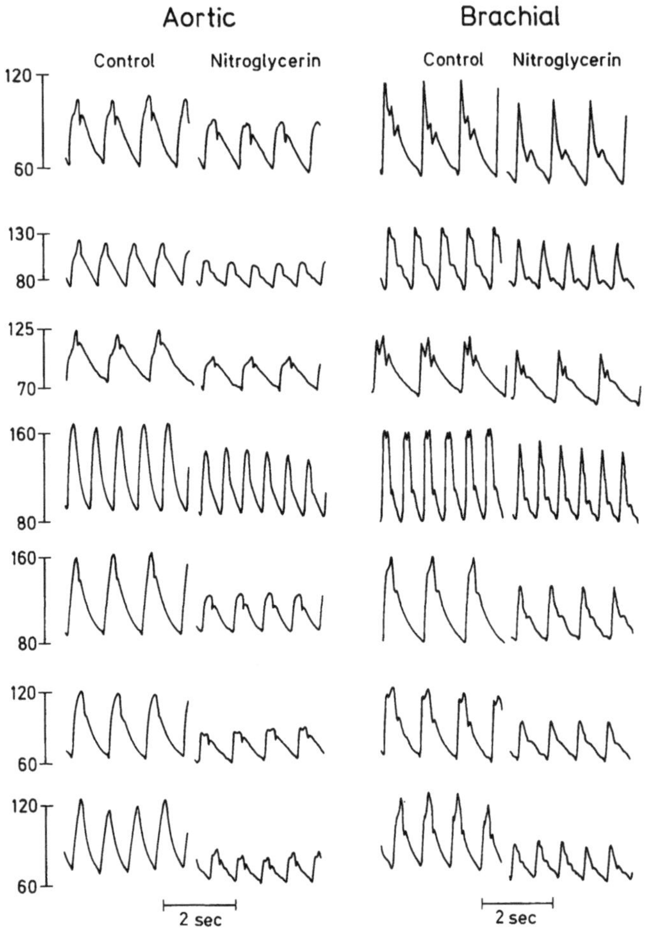

Fig. 7 (Left panel): Pressure waves recorded in the ascending aorta of 14 patients before (left) and after (right) administration of nitroglycerin 0.3 mg sublingually. (Right panel): Pressure waves in the brachial artery of the same patients before (left) and after (right) administration of nitroglycerin. There were consistent and sub-

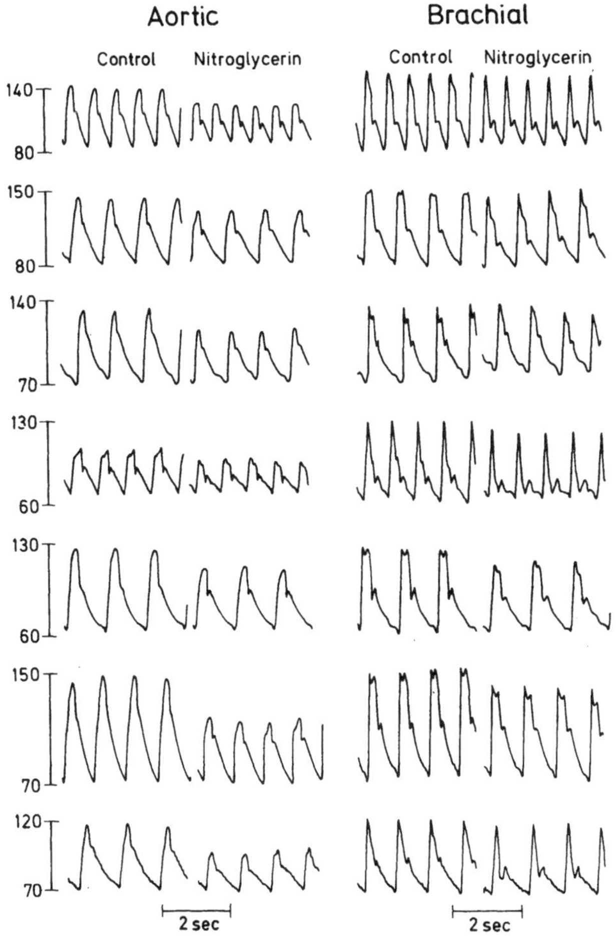

stantial falls in aortic systolic pressure (averaging 22.2 mm Hg) but inconsistent and lesser falls in brachial systolic pressure (averaging 11.9 mm Hg). From Kelly et al. [12].

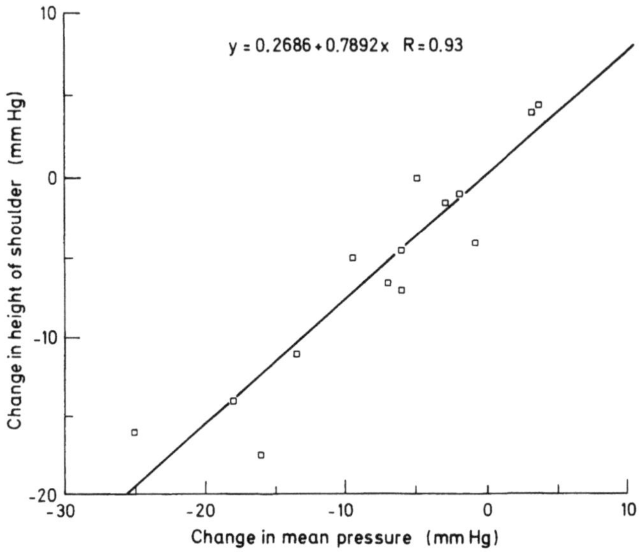

Fig. 8 Relationship between change in height to the systolic shoulder of pressure in the ascending aorta (X in fig. 1) to change in mean pressure following nitroglycerin therapy in the 14 patients illustrated in fig. 7. From Kelly et al. [12].

patients, nitroglycerin always caused a greater reduction in ascending aortic than brachial artery systolic pressure. Sometimes, brachial systolic pressure did not fall at all even when aortic systolic pressure fell by 20 mm Hg (fig. 1). Overall, the brachial systolic pressure fall with nitroglycerin was 10.3 mm Hg less than the fall in aortic systolic pressure (fig. 7). In the whole series of patients, mean pressure fell by 7.5 mm Hg; this was attributed to concurrent venodilation with reduction in stroke volume without change in peripheral resistance. This explanation was enhanced by finding of a linear relationship between fall in mean pressure to the reduction in pressure rise to the first systolic shoulder in the ascending aorta (fig. 8).

These findings for nitroglycerin appear to apply to other agents which cause arterial or arteriolar dilation with consequent decrease in wave reflection from peripheral sites. Nitroglycerin however appears to be the most potent drug to decrease wave reflection acutely, and possibly the only such drug to reduce wave reflection without decreasing peripheral resistance. In non invasive studies, dilevalol [11] has been shown to decrease systolic pressure in central arteries to a greater degree than in the radial artery. In a recent study Simkus et al. [7]

have shown at cardiac catheterisation, similar differential affects of nitroprusside on aortic and brachial pressures to those we have shown for nitroglycerin.

The recent studies summarised here [11–15, 25] represent the culmination of about 30 years work on arterial hemodynamics.

They appear to show:

1. That in mature adult humans, wave reflection causes substantial augmentation of ascending aortic and left ventricular systolic pressure without corresponding augmentation of pressure in the brachial or radial artery.
2. That nitroglycerin, through reduction in wave reflection, causes substantial reduction in ascending aortic and left ventricular systolic pressure without corresponding reduction in brachial and radial pressure.
3. That nitroglycerin is an effective and potent agent for reduction in left ventricular after load, but whose effects are underestimated from conventional measurements of arterial pressure in the brachial artery.
4. That changes in arterial pressure and left ventricular load can be studied noninvasively with the new technique of applanation tonometry.

These studies are complementary to other reports and are not inconsistent with any known data.

We in Sydney are currently seeking ways for better analysis of the arterial pulse as recorded invasively in the brachial or radial artery or noninvasively in the radial artery by applanation tonometry. We seek to complement conventional pressure recordings of systolic and diastolic pressure so as to better understand the subtle affects of nitroglycerin and other vasoactive agents on left ventricular load. From change in peripheral pulse contour we can infer beneficial or detrimental effects on left ventricular load [25]. This approach harks back to earlier times before the ubiquitous brachial cuff sphygmomanometer was introduced, and when clinical information on hypertension and other diseases was determined from study of the arterial pulse by sphygmography [10].

References

[1] Avolio, A. P., Chen Shang-Gong, Wang Ruo-Ping et al.: Effects of aging on changing arterial compliance and left ventricular load in a northern Chinese urban community. Circulation *68* (1983) 50–58.

[2] Avolio, A. P., Deng Fa-Quan, Li Wei-Quiang et al.: Effects of aging on arterial distensibility in populations with high and low prevalence of hypertension: comparison between urban and rural communities in China. Circulation *71* (1985) 202–210.

[3] Bramwell, J. V., A. V. Hill: Velocity of transmission of the pulse wave and elasticicty of arteries. Lancet *1* (1922) 891 – 892.
[4] Brown, B. G., E. Bolson, R. B. Peterson et al.: The mechanisms of nitroglycerin action: stenosis vasodilation as a major component of the drug response. Circulation *64* (1981) 1089 – 1097.
[5] Feldman, R. L., C. J. Pepine, C. R. Conti: Magnitude of dilation of large and small coronary arteries by nitroglycerin. Circualtion *64* (1981) 324 – 333.
[6] Fitchett, D.: The effects of nitroglycerin on forearm arterial compliance. J. Clin. Invest. Med. *5* (Suppl.) (1982) 31.
[7] Simkus, G. J., D. H. Fitchett: Radial arterial pressure measurements may be a poor guide to the beneficial effects of nitroprusside on left ventricular systolic pressure in congestive heart failure. Am. J. Cardio. *66* (1990) 323 – 326.
[8] Fitchett, D. H., G. J. Simkus, J. P. Beaudry et al.: Reflected pressure waves in the ascending aorta: effect of glyceryl trinitrate. Cardiovasc. Res. *22* (1988) 494 – 500.
[9] Hugenholtz, P. G., D. G. Julian: International symposium: nitrates, 1987. Eur. Heart. J. *9* (Suppl. A) (1988).
[10] Karamanoglu, M., R. Kelly, G. Gravalee et al.: Clinical implications of pressure wave transmission in the upper limb. Circulation *80* (Suppl. 2) (1989) 542.
[11] Kelly, R., J. Daley, A. P. Avolio et al.: Arterial dilation and reduced wave reflection. Benefit of Dilevalol in Hypertension. Hypertension *14* (1989) 14 – 21.
[12] Kelly, R. P., H. H. Gibbs, M. F. O'Rourke et al.: Nitroglycerin has more favourable effects on left ventricular afterload than apparent from measurement of pressure in a peripheral artery. Eur. Heart J. *11* (1990) 138 – 144.
[13] Kelly, R., C. Hayward, A. P. Avolio et al.: Non invasive determination of age-related changes in the human arterial pulse. Circulation *80* (1989) 1652 – 1659.
[14] Kelly, R., C. Hayward, J. Ganis et al.: Non invasive registration of the arterial pressure pulse waveform using high-fidelity applanation tonometry. J. Vasc. Med. Biol. *1* (Suppl. 3) (1989) 142 – 149.
[15] Kelly, R., M. Karamanoglu, H. Gibbs et al.: Noninvasive carotid pressure wave registration as an indicator of ascending aortic pressure. J. Vasc. Med. Biol. *1* (Suppl. 4) (1989) 241 – 247
[16] Latson, T. W., W. C. Hunter, N. Katoh et al.: Effect of nitroglycerin on aortic impedance, diameter, and pulse wave velocity. Circ. Res. *62* (1988) 884 – 890.
[17] McDonald, D. A.: Blood flow in arteries. Arnold, London 1960.
[18] McDonald, D. A., M. G. Taylor: The hydrodynamics of the arterial circulation. Progress in Biophysics *9* (1959) 107 – 173.
[19] McGregor, M.: The nitrates and myocardial ischaemia. Circulation *66* (1982) 689 – 692.
[20] Mills C. J., I. T. Gabe, J. H. Gault et al.: Pressure-flow relationships and vascular impedance in man. Cardiovasc. Res. *4* (1970) 405 – 417.
[21] Murgo, J. P., N. Westerhof, J. P. Giolma et al.: Aortic input impedance in normal man: relationship to pressure wave forms. Circulation *62* (1980) 105 – 116.
[22] O'Rourke, M. F.: Pressure and flow in systemic arteries and the anatomical design of the arterial system. J. Appl. Physio. *23* (1967) 139 – 149.

[23] O'Rourke, M. F.: Arterial haemodynamics in hypertension. Cir. Res. *26* u. *27* (11) (1970) 123–133.
[24] O'Rourke, M. F. Arterial Function in Health and Disease. Churchill, Edinburgh 1982.
[25] O'Rourke, M. F. What is blood pressure? Am. J. Hypertension *3* (1990) 803–810.
[26] O'Rourke, M. F., A. P. Avolio: Pulsatile flow and pressure in human systemic arteries: studies in man and in a multi-branched model of the human systemic arterial tree. Cir. Res. *46* (3) (1980) 363–372.
[27] O'Rourke, M. F., J. V. Blazek, C. L. Morreels jr. et al.: Pressure wave transmission along the human aorta: changes with age and in arterial degenerative disease. Cir. Res. *23* (1968) 567–579.
[28] O'Rourke, M. F., R. P. Kelly, A. P. Avolio et al.: Effects of arterial dilator agents on central aortic systolic pressure and on left ventricular hydraulic load. Am. J. Cardiol. *63* (1989) 381–441.
[29] O'Rourke, M. F., M. G. Taylor: Vascular impedance of the systemic circulation. Cir. Res. *18* (1966) 126–139.
[30] O'Rourke, M. F., M. G. Taylor: Input impedance of the systemic circulation. Cir. Res. *20* (1967) 365–380.
[31] Parmely, W. W.: Medical treatment of congestive heart failure. Where are we now? Circulation *75* (Suppl. 4) (1987) 4–10.
[32] Roy, C. S.: The elastic properties of the arterial wall. J. Physio. (London) *3* (1880) 125–159.
[33] Rutherford, J. D., E. Braunwald, P. Cohn: Chronic ischaemic heart disease. In: E. Braunwald (Ed.): Heart Disease, pp. 1327–1328. W. B. Saunders, Philadelphia 1988.
[34] Simon, A. C., J. A. Levenson, B. I. Levi et al.: Effect of nitroglycerin on peripheral large arteries in hypertension. Br. J. Clin. Pharmacol. *14* (1982) 241–246.
[35] Smith, T. W., E. Braunwald, R. A. Kelly: The management of heart failure. In: E. Braunwald (Ed.): Heart Disease 3rd. edn., pp. 516–523. W. B. Saunders, Philadelphia 1988.
[36] Takazawa, K.: A clinical study of the second component of left systolic pressure. J. Tokyo Medical College *45* (1987) 256–270.
[37] Taylor, M. G.: An approach to an analysis of the arterial pulse wave. I Oscillations in an attenuating line. Phys. Med. Biol. *1* (1957a) 258–269.
[38] Taylor, M. G.: An approach to an analysis of the arterial pulse wave. II Fluid oscillations in an elastic tube. Phys. Med. Biol. *1* (1957b) 321–329.
[39] Taylor, M. G.: Wave travel in arteries and the design of the cardiovascular system. In: E. O. Attinger (Ed.): Pulsatile Blood Flow, pp. 343–372. McGraw Hill, New York 1963.
[40] Taylor, M. G.: The input impedance of an assembly of randomly branching elastic tubes. Biophysical J. *6* (1966) 29–51.
[41] Taylor, M. G.: The elastic properties of arteries in relation to the physiological functions of the arterial system. Gastroenterology *52* (1967) 358–363.
[42] Yaginuma, T., A. P. Avolio, M. F. O'Rourke et al.: Effect of glyceryl nitrate on peripheral arteries alters left ventricular hydrualic load in man. Cardiovasc. Res. *20* (1986) 153–160.

[43] Westling, H., L. Jansson, B. Jonson et al.: Vasoactive drugs and elastic properties of human arteries in vivo, with special reference to the action of nitroglycerin. Eur. Heart. J. *5* (1984) 609–616.
[44] Womersley, J. R.: The mathematical analysis of the arterial circulation in a state of oscillatory motion. Wright Air Development Center, Technical Report WADC-TR56-614, 1958.
[45] Womersley, J. R.: Oscillatory flow in arteries: the reflection of the pulse wave at junctions and rigid inserts in the arterial system. Phys. Med. Biol. *2* (1958) 313–323.

Nitroglycerin in the therapy of acute myocardial infarction

W.-D. Bussmann

Introduction

When we began first testing the action of nitroglycerin in recent cardiac infarction in 1972, the substance was still considered contra-indicated for use in the acute infarction phase. A rise in heart rate and sharp fall in blood pressure was feared. The first systematic investigations in Frankfurt (1974), however, showed that nitroglycerin has very definite positive hemodynamic effects on recent cardiac infarction, especially in patients with left ventricular failure [4, 5]. Chiche et al. [11] have performed investigations on the effects of nitroglycerin in France, and reported their results in 1978/79 [11, 12]. In spite of the work of Flaherty et al. [14] in 1975, the use of the new therapy in the United States has not become widespread. Sodium nitroprusside has long been preferred there. Judgutt et al. [15, 16] demonstrated, first in experimental, then in larger clinical trials, that nitroglycerin has a more beneficial effect in the treatment of infarction (1981/82).

In German-speaking countries, the prescription of intravenous nitroglycerin has been practically obligatory for many years. Now the United States is also turning towards the routine use of nitroglycerin in recent infarction cases. This was made public in a 1990 therapy recommendation of the American College of Cardiology and the American Heart Association in the Journal Circulation, AHA Medical/Scientific Statement [1]. According to the collection of publications dealing with the use of nitroglycerin in infarction cases published by Yusuf [20], it was once again made clear that nitroglycerin can reduce the infarction size and, possibly, have a positive effect on the prognosis. The statement of the American Cardiologic Society has therefore recommended nitroglycerin as a primary medication in the treatment of infarction. A reduction in infarction size and protection from ventricular fibrillation can be expected in most patients, when used during the onset of symptoms and when systolic blood pressure values decreases not below 90 mm Hg. Prolonged infusion is indicated with thrombolytic therapy. Our own findings dealing with this topic will be discussed below.

Mechanism of action

Some important new experimental and clinical findings have recently allowed the mechanism of action of nitroglycerin to appear in a new light. The fact that nitroglycerin dilatates the epicardial coronary arteries has been supplemented by the recent findings of Feldman et al. [13] which show that nitroglycerin is able to expand narrowed segments of the epicardial coronary arteries. This results in a marked rise in flow into the ischemic area. We were able to show that even minimal doses of nitroglycerin cause a dilatation of coronary stenosis while neither sinking filling pressure, decreasing arterial blood pressure nor dilating segments of the undiseased coronary artery. This effect partially explains the antianginal efficacy of nitroglycerin [10, 18, 19].

It is known from the systematic investigations performed by Hess et al. [15] and from our own measurements, that during an angina-pectoris attack the epicardial coronary arteries contract strongly. This is probably also the case in acute myocardial infarction.

Vasoconstricting elements apparently prevail. Increased renin-angiotensin and alpha-receptor-stimulators contribute to vasoconstriction, particularly because the Endothelial Derived Relaxing Factor (EDRF) has no effect on defective intima. Through the contraction of the coronary arteries, particularly in the stenotic areas, the rate of flow is further decreased and myocardial ischemia increased. Shear force and irrigation effect decrease, promoting the formation of thrombus. This mechanism also possibly provides the explanation for the fact that the extent of the infarction is frequently much larger in juveniles than is indicated by the perfusion area of the closed vessel.

The application of nitroglycerin results in the dilatation of the contracted coronary vessel system. Nitroglycerin replaces the missing EDRF in the defective intima through the release of nitrous oxide (NO) (Bassenge [3]). This results in dilatation, particularly of contracted vascular sections. In some cases incompletely occluded segments can be freed. The resulting rise in flow produces an irrigating effect, and fewer thrombocytes are thus able to be deposited in the area of the stenosed segment. In addition, nitroglycerin has an antiaggregating effect [2].

It therefore follows that the local effects of nitroglycerin on the coronary arteries are much more marked than the better-known peripheral effects. It was earlier assumed that the beneficial anti-ischemic effect of nitroglycerin was a result of relief in the peripheral areas through venous and arterial vasodilatation. The direct coronary effect was rejected. Today the opinion has been reversed. The local coronary effects, i. e. the distension of coronary stenosis, is the main factor in the improvement of circulation in the ischemic area.

It is also possible that the interruption of an anginal attack by nitroglycerin is primarily a result of the improvement in circulation into the affected vascular areas, whereby the peripheral effects on circulation certainly have a complementary effect.

Venous pooling is especially important in patients with cardiac infarction and left ventricular failure. Congestion can be halved within 3 minutes through the displacement of 200 – 250 ml of blood. The filling pressure frequently decreases by 50%, which also results in an improvement in endocardial circulation. This further promotes myocardial contraction in the affected areas and improves output capacity.

A decrease in blood pressure is caused by the distension of the arterioles through a drop in peripheral resistance. This also causes a rise in cardiac output in patients with cardiac failure. The increase in cardiac output can be brought about solely through improved flow into the affected myocardium if more blood reaches the ischemic area through the dilatation of the coronary stenosis.

These specific findings about the mechanism of action of nitroglycerin probably have considerable significance in the beneficial treatment of myocardial ischemia in an acute infarction situation. The dilatation of the stenosis diameter by nitroglycerin is of decided importance for the further development and distension of the infarction.

In the much more frequently occuring complete occlusion, the effect of nitroglycerin hinders the development to total infarction through the improvement in collateral circulation, which has been proven under treatment with nitroglycerin.

In addition, the dilatation of stenosis in arteries not affected by the infarction can also have a beneficial effect on the magnitude of the infarction. Spontaneous or medical thrombolysis is probably more effective in the presence of nitroglycerin. The dilatation of the stenosis at the root of the occlusion can accelerate the thrombolytic process. The antiaggregating effect of nitroglycerin may possibly hinder a reocclusion. The increased flow in the coronary area can be improved by the effect of the shear force and irrigation effect on thrombocytes or thrombotic material.

Our studies on 60 patients showed a significant reduction in the CK- and CK-MB-infarction size, a decrease in myocardial ischemia measured at the ST-segment, and a reduction of the QRS-necrosis signs in the EKG. The ischemic ventricular arrythmias decreased [6, 7, 8]. It could also be concluded from the investigations that patients who received nitroglycerin initially had a lower early mortality rate and a better late prognosis than the patients in the control group [9].

It must be added, that during the first two deciding days of infarction, small dosages of intravenously administered nitroglycerin do not lead to a reduction of the effect on the left-ventricular filling pressure. The 2-day-long uninterrupted infusion of nitroglycerin in the case of recent infarction can thus be considered standard therapy.

References

[1] AHA Medical/Scientific Statement: ACC/AHA Guidelines for the Early Management of Patients With Acute Myocardial Infarction. Circulation *82* (1990) 664–707.

[2] Bassenge, E., H. Gauch: Stellenwert von EDRF als Mediator der Gefäßregulation. Einfluß des Gefäßendothels auf den vaskulären Tonus und die Thrombozytenfunktion. Fortschr. Med. *106* (1988) 44–46.

[3] Bassenge, E.: Experimentelle Befunde zur Nitratwirkung. In: H. Roskamm (Hrsg.): Nitroglycerin VI, pp. 53–66. Walter de Gruyter, Berlin–New York 1989.

[4] Bussmann, W. D., J. Vachalowa, M. Kaltenbach: Wirkung von Nitroglycerin beim frischen Herzinfarkt (Abstract). Z. Kardiol. *52* (Suppl. I) (1974a) 63.

[5] Bussmann, W. D., J. Löhner, M. Kaltenbach: Orale Nitroglycerinpräparate in der Behandlung der Linksinsuffizienz beim frischen Herzinfarkt (Abstract). Z. Kardiol. *52* (Suppl. I) (1974b) 63.

[6] Bussmann, W. D., H. Schöfer, M. Kaltenbach: Wirkung von Nitroglycerin beim akuten Myocardinfarkt. II. Intravenöse Dauerinfusion von Nitroglycerin bei Patienten mit und ohne Linksinsuffizienz und ihre Auswirkung auf die Infarktgröße. Dtsch. Med. Wschr. *101* (1976) 642–648.

[7] Bussmann, W. D., D. Passek, W. Seidel et al.: Reduktion der CK- und CK-MB-Enzymaktivität und der Infarktgröße durch intravenöses Nitroglycerin. Z. Kardiol. *69* (1980) 18–30.

[8] Bussmann, W. D., D. Passek, W. Seidel et al.: Reduction of CK and CK-MB indexes of infarct size by intravenous nitroglycerin. Circulation *63* (1981) 615–622.

[9] Bussmann, W. D., M. Haller: Hinweis auf eine Abnahme der Früh- und Spätmortalität beim frischen Herzinfarkt unter Nitroglycerintherapie. Klin. Wochenschr. *61* (1983) 417–422.

[10] Bussmann, W. D.: Transdermal nitroglycerin: Concluding remarks. In: W. D. Bussmann, A. Zanchetti (Hrsg.): Transdermal nitroglycerin therapy, pp. 66–71. Hans Huber Publishers, Berlin–Stuttgart Toronto 1985.

[11] Chiche, P., S. J. Baligadoo, J. P. Derrida: A randomised trial of prolonged nitroglycerin infusion in acute myocardial infarction (Abstract). Circulation *59/60* (Suppl. II) (1979) 165.

[12] Derrida, J. P., R. Sal, P. Gliche: Favorable effects of prolonged nitroglycerin infusion in patients with acute myocardial infarction. Am. Heart J. *96* (1978) 833–834.

[13] Feldmann, R. L., C. J. Pepine, C. R. Conti: Magnitude of dilatation of large and small coronary arteries by nitroglycerin. Circulation *64* (1981) 324–333.

[14] Flaherty, J.T., P. R. Reid, D.T. Kelly et al.: Intravenous nitroglycerin in acute myocardial infarction. Circulation *51* (1975) 132–139.
[15] Hess, O. M., A. Bortone, K. Eid et al.: Coronary vasomotor tone during static and dynamic exercise. Eur. Heart. J. *10* (Suppl. F) (1990) 105–110.
[16] Jugdutt, B. I., L. C. Becker, G. M. Hutchins et al.: Effect of intravenous nitroglycerin on collateral blood flow and infarct size in the concious dog. Circulation *63* (1981) 17–28.
[17] Jugdutt, B. I., B. A. Sussex, J.W. Warnica: Persistent reduction in left ventricular asynergy in acute myocardial infarction with intravenous nitroglycerin infusion (Abstract). Circulation *66* (Suppl. II) (1982) 2.
[18] Sievert, H., W. Rimili, W. Schneider et al.: Antianginöse Wirksamkeit minimaler Nitroglycerindosen. Z. Kardiol. *74* (Suppl. III) (1985) 80.
[19] Sievert, H., G. Selzer, G. Kober et al.: Nitroglycerin intravenös in extrem niedriger Dosierung bewirkt eine Erweiterung von Koronarstenosen. Z. Kardiol. *76* (Suppl. I) (1987) 272.
[20] Yusuf, S., S. MacMahon, R. Collins et al.: Effect of intravenous nitrates on mortality in acute myocardial infarction: an overview of the randomised trails. The Lancet (1988) 1088–1092.

Clinical findings in the treatment of hypertensive crisis with nitroglycerin

H. P. Nast

Introduction

As a result of its myocardial, coronary and cerebral effects as well as its effect on kidney function, a hypertensive crisis represents an immediate vital danger to the patient and can lead to death within only a few hours [1]. The main complications are hypertensive encephalopathy, intercranial bleeding, acute myocardial infarction, pulmonary edema with left ventricular insufficiency, secreting aneurisms and acute kidney failure. Cardiac complications occur particularly frequently during a hypertensive crisis. 50–80% of patients with hypertony exhibit previous cardiac damages [5]. In addition, patients with coronary heart disease with an excessive rise in blood pressure exhibit inferior hemodynamic prospects.

The definition of a hypertensive crisis is not bound by specific blood pressure limits [5]. The deciding factor is not the absolute blood pressure level but the dynamics and extent of the rise in blood pressure, the initial blood pressure and previous damages to the cardiovascular system.

Particular danger to the patient occurs when the excessive rise in blood pressure strikes an insufficiently adapted vascular system. This is the case when a sudden rise in blood pressure originates from a normal or only slightly higher blood pressure condition. On the other hand, an excessively high blood pressure of, for example, 270/120 mmHg does not represent a hypertensive crisis for patients with known severe or malignant hypertonia.

There are few conditions of illness which demand such quick therapy as the hypertensive crisis in order to prevent irreparable damages or, as the case may be, lethal consequences.

In the case of a hypertensive emergency, the immediate and effective lowering of the blood pressure takes preference over all further diagnostic measures. Because of the rapid progression of vascular-dependent damage, the degree of reversibility of complications is directly related to the speed with which effective treatment is begun. Therapy should therefore be initiated before admission to the hospital. A lowering of systolic blood pressure to 130–160 mmHg and of diastolic blood pressure to approximately 100–110 mmHg is necessary and sufficient. A decrease in the blood pressure should occur within a few minutes. It should be noted however, that a drastic lowering of blood pressure within a very short time by means of intravenous administration of antihypertensives may cause problems and can have, in certain circumstances, dire consequences [4]. A moderate lowering of the blood pressure is then necessary when ischemic symptoms of the brain and heart appear or worsen. Particular care must be observed in older patients and in patients with carotid stenoses. The reliability of a medically induced decrease in blood pressure is of vital necessity in a hypertensive crisis. Antihypertensives used in therapy of a hypertensive crisis should work quickly and reliably in lowering blood pressure, should be easily controllable and should have minimal side effects. In the past, reserpine, cloridine, dihydralazine, sodium nitroprusside and dioxide were employed as emergency antihypertensives. Nevertheless, these therapeutical possibilities resulted in part in unpleasant and sometimes serious side effects. Because of its generally uncomplicated application and controllability, the calcium antagonist nifedipine, an orally ingestible substance, or the alphablocker, ebrantil, have been the treatment of choice over the above-named medicines for the past several years for parenteral application.

When considering the cardiovascular complications in a hypertensive crisis, such as acute left ventrical failure, pulmonary edema, angina pectoris or impending myocardial infarction, nitroglycerin presents itself as the ideal emergency medication. In addition to the known effects of nitrate which include dilation of the postcapillary vascular segment with a decrease in the venous reflux, a sinking of the pulmonary capillary pressure, and a diminution of the enddiastolic pressure in the left ventricle, a dilation of the large arterial vessels, which in turn leads to a decrease in blood pressure, after-load, cardiac activity and myocardial oxygen consumption occurs.

The antihypertensive effect of nitroglycerin in a hypertensive crisis was first submitted by Rupp during the second Nitroglycerin Symposium in Hamburg in 1979 [8]. An easily controllable, careful, sufficient lowering of crisis-induced high blood pressure could be attained using both oral and parenteral application. However, because of the fact that the sublingual administration of nifedipine is still preferred in general out-patient treatment of hypertensive crisis, especially in the pre-hospital phase, a comparative study of nitroglycerin, likewise applied in sublingual form, presented itself. First, a five-part crossover study with increasing dosages of nifedipine and nitroglycerin was carried out in order to determine equipotent doses of the two medications. After a reasonable measure of agreement was reached between 10 mg of nifedipine, and 1.2 mg of nitroglycerin (Nitrolingual® forte), the antihypertensive efficacy and tolerance of Nitrolingual® forte was tested against that of nifedipine in the treatment of excessive high blood pressure, with or without clinical symptoms in a multicentered, open, random study.

Method

This study was carried out in five clinical centers: Bussmann (coord.), Nast, Kenedi, von Mengden and Rachor. The trial was carried out on a total of 40 patients ages 46–85, who were required to exhibit the following criteria: systolic blood pressure of at least 185 mmHg and diastolic blood pressure of at least 105 mmHg. Blood pressure upon admission to the study was, on average, systolic, 210.5 mmHg and diastolic, 115.3 mmHg. Men made up 37.5% and women, 62.5% of the study population. The median duration of hypertonia was 9 years, and an excessive high pressure in the anamnesis occurred in 47.5% of the patients.

Eight patients were recruited in each center. Four patients with cardiac and/or cerebral symptoms were assigned to Group A under the category "Hypertensive crisis," and four patients, with excessive increase in blood pressure but without clinical symptoms were assigned to Group B. Within groups A and B, 2 patients were treated in random succession with nifedipine with 10 mg capsules and with nitroglycerin in the form of Nitrolingual® forte with 1.2 mg capsules. The nifedipine capsule was bitten through and the contents were swallowed immediately afterwards with a little fluid. The nitroglycerin capsule was likewise bitten through. The patient allowed the contents of the capsule to dissolve in the oral cavity.

Blood pressure, pulse rate, and cardial and cerebral symptoms were recorded 3 minutes, 5 minutes and 10 minutes after the administration of the capsule. When a normalisation of blood pressure was not achieved within 10 minutes of the first administration, a second application of the test medication was given. The second application consisted of a double dosage. That is, if the first application consisted of Nitrolingual® forte, the patient received Nitrolingual® forte again in the second application. Further controls were effected 13, 15, 20, 45 and 60 minutes, as well as 1, 2, 4 and 6 hours after the first application.

The target parameters were the systolic and diastolic blood pressure and, in Group A, the cardiac and/or cerebral signs and symptoms of the hypertensive crisis.

Statistical evaluation was performed according to the Chi-Square-test and the t-test for related random samples, and with variance-analysis of repeated measures.

Results

In 27 cases, the patients was being admitted to the hospital. 13 cases dealt with hospitalised patients. In 17 cases, whereby 10 patients received Nitrolingual® and 7 nifedipine, the single application sufficed. A second application was necessary after 10 minutes in 10 cases in the Nitrolingual® group and in 13 cases in the nifedipine group.

An average reduction in systolic blood pressure after 3 minutes from 210.9 mmHg over 180.1 mmHg to 168.5 mmHg after 10 minutes was observed after the first application of Nitrolingual® forte. A weak initial reduction in systolic blood pressure from 210.2 mmHg over 196.9 mmHg after 3 minutes to 174.3 mmHg after 10 minutes occurred after the application of nifedipine (fig. 1). Thereafter, an initial and significantly stronger reduction of systolic blood pressure under Nitrolingual® forte than under nifedipine was observed. This could be confirmed by the test of parallelity of the curves (fig. 2). The diastolic blood pressure showed a parallel decrease in both preparation groups, under

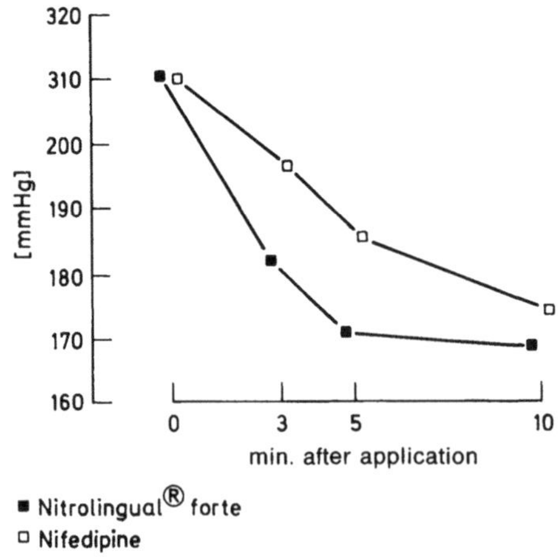

Fig. 1 Average values of systolic blood pressure up to 10 min. after application of Nitrolingual® forte or nifedipine.

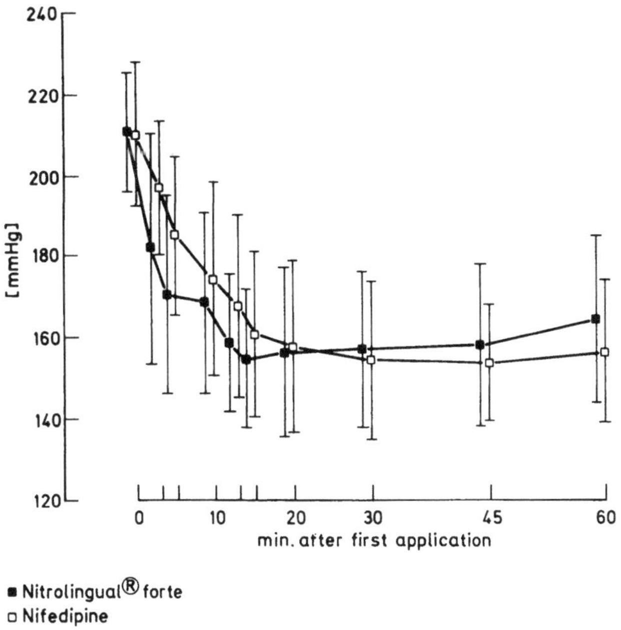

Fig. 2 Average values and standard deviations of systolic blood pressure up to 60 minutes after application of Nitrolingual® forte or nifedipine.

Nitrolingual® forte on average from 112.4 mmHg to 94.8 mmHg and under nifedipine from 118.3 mmHg to 99.5 mmHg after 10 minutes. No conspicuous changes in pulse rate were demonstrated.

After the second application of Nitrolingual® forte (Nitrolingual® forte: N = 10, nifedipine: n = 13), a renewed reduction in the systolic blood pressure occurred in the Nitrolingual group. In addition, the diastolic pressure also decreased more strongly 3 minutes after the application.

The differences in systolic and diastolic blood pressure remained on the whole, however, statistically borderline values.

While during the continuous, blood pressure-lowering effect up to one hour after the first application, no particular differences were noted in either of the test groups of Nitrolingual® forte and nifedipine, statistically insignificant decreases in systolic blood pressure were observed under nifedipine. Ultimately, in the course of up to 6 hours, no significant differences between the two groups were observed (fig. 3).

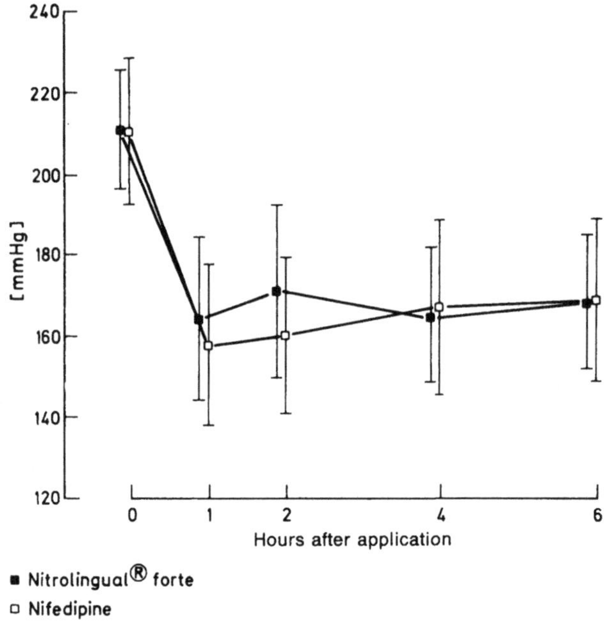

Fig. 3 Average values and standard deviations in systolic blood pressure up to 6 hours after application of Nitrolingual® forte or nifedipine.

No fundamental differences were observed between the two groups with respect to an improvement in the symptoms with regards to the influence on cardial and cerebral symptoms during the hypertensive crisis.

Undesirable medicinal effects occurred in two cases after the use of Nitrolingual® forte and in 4 cases after nifedipine. Seen as a whole, the antihypertensive effect and compatibility of both preparations was comparatively good.

Summary

These results demonstrate the sound therapeutic efficacy of nitroglycerin in lowering blood pressure in cases of hypertensive crisis and of excessive rise in blood pressure. On the whole, nitroglycerin has, in comparison with nifedipine, an initially stronger antihypertensive effect, which naturally serves the goal of the therapy: to lower blood pressure as quickly as possible. In agreement with the results of other researchers, the systolic blood pressure is more sharply lowered than the diastolic. This causes the main effect to be registered within the first 10 minutes of application [2, 8]. The effect remains, remarkably, for up to 6 hours. The efficient decrease in blood pressure with nitroglycerin is not only a result of the decrease in afterload through the direct effect on the peripheral resistance vessels, but also of the simultaneous dilation of the peripheral capacity vessels with an increase of venous pooling, through which the blood supply, or pre-load to the heart decreases. Correspondingly, heart filling, myocardial wall tension and cardial volume decrease and the blood pressure is lowered [3, 7]. The advantages of nitroglycerin are, in contrast to nifedipine, its ability to quickly limit the impending danger of acute left ventrical failure or pulmonary edema, and in the case of previously existing coronary heart-disease, to hinder angina pectoris, or myocardial infarction. Thus, nitroglycerin therapy with nitroglycerin sublingual in a dosage of 1.2 mg of Nitrolingual® forte, should be commenced in out-patient emergency treatment before admission to a hospital.

References

[1] Aken von, H. et al.: Hochdruckkrise – Lebensbedrohliche Komplikationen erfordern rasches Handeln. Intensiv Care. *9* (1983) 123.

[2] Bussmann, W. D., J. Vachalowa, M. Kaltenbach: Die Wirkung von Nitroglycerin beim akuten Myocardinfarkt. Dtsch. Med. Wschr. *14* (1975) 749.

[3] Hagemann, K., B. Niehus, G. Arnold et al.: Intravasales Volumen und Strömungswiderstand des großen und kleinen Kreislaufs unter Wirkung von Nitroglycerin. Verhandlungen Deutsche Gesellschaft für Kreislaufforschung *39* (1973) 243.

[4] Klaus, D.: Akute hypertensive Encephalopathie. Diagnostik und Therapie. Intensiv. med. *20* (1983) 45.

[5] Lang, R., W. Kaufmann: Prinzipielle Diagnostik bei Hochdruckkrankheit. Intensiv. med. *20* (1983) 199.

[6] Nast, H. P.: Hypertensive Krise: Nitroglycerin oder Nifedipin-Kapseln geben? Therapiewoche *38* (1986) 3896.

[7] Raff, W. K., W. Lochner: Wirkungsmechanismus von Nitroglycerin. Med. Klin. *25* (1974) 1100.

[8] Rupp, M., H. Scherrer, H. P. Lutz et al.: Nitroglycerin bei hypertensiver Krise. In: Zweites Hamburger Nitroglycerin-Symposion 1979, p. 87. Pharmazeutische Verlagsgesellschaft, München 1979.

The treatment of renal colics with glycerol trinitrate

M. Kriegmair, A. Hofstetter

Introduction

For years, the routine treatment of colic-like pains associated with nephrolithiasis has been combination preparations containing metamizole. As a result of the Federal Health Authority's (Bundesgesundheitsamt) withdrawal of the registration for combination preparations containing metamizole, the discussion concerning alternative treatment possibilities has been provoked once again [1]. Randomized comparative studies on this problem have not been presented to date. The application of opioids should be reserved for severe conditions of pain and can only be applied after definite diagnosis. Apart from that, the danger exists that conditions of pain, produced by an acute abdomen, may be concealed. The further differential diagnostics, which for most part rely upon the clinical examination, would be confounded by an early application of opioids. The prostaglandin synthesis inhibitor and antirheumatic agents such as diclofenac-sodium have proven successful in the prophylaxis of recurrent ureteral colics. In the event of acute pain, however, they are less suited because of their delayed onset of action. The ureteral colic is interpreted primarily as a dilating pain. Under these conditions, a spasmolytic agent with a prompt onset of action would be desirable. Nitroglycerin has proven to be such a spasmolytic agent for years in the treatment of coronary heart disease. After intracellular conversion to nitrosothiol, nitroglycerin results in the extracellular discharge of calcium. The reduction of intracellular calcium concentrations produces a relaxation of the non-striated musculature. This spasmolytic treatment serves not only the cardiovascular system but also the non-striated musculature of the ureter leading to an evident increase in the pressure and pain tolerance of internal dilatation, as shown in the clinical investigations by Dunzendorfer [2].

Comparatively, glycerol trinitrate has been successfully employed as a biliary colic spasmolytic as well as a premedication in ERPC for years [3].

Considering this background it would seem legitimate to submit glycerol trinitrate to clinical testing for ureteral colics as well. A previous study of dosage levels from Dunzendorfer showed that the known cardiological dosage did not reach an adequate spasmolytic effect [2]. 0.8 and 1.2 mg glycerol trinitrate parenterally injected proved ineffective. With 1.6 mg as well, only a slight alleviation of pain could be attained. The pain intensity was reduced to half of its average, original level only after increasing the dosage to 2.4 mg.

In December, 1987 we began an open, randomized, clinical trial with Nitrolingual® forte capsules versus Nitrolingual®-Spray versus Nitro Pohl® infus versus butylscopalaminbromide i. v. The goal of this trial was to establish in which respect a treatment with glycerol trinitrate, in terms of comparative efficacy and toxicity would be comparable to a standard treatment and which form of administration – spray, capsules, or i. v. injection – would be considered optimal.

Patients and methods

A total of 80 patients were submitted to a block randomization. The individual treatment groups included 20 patients each. One patient of the butylscopolaminbromide group had to be excluded because the randomization of the patient occurred twice. The total collective had an average age of 51.2 years; the youngest patient was 22, the oldest patient was 80. 32% presented with a ureteral colic which had been treated with extracorporal shock wave lithotripsy, and in 68% the treatment occurred because of an acute spontaneous ureteral colic.

In 16.5% a lithiasis of the renal pelvis and calix as basic illness was present and in 83.5% a ureterolithiasis. 57.7% of the patients were treated for a recurrent colic. Among the trial groups there existed no pronounced, statistical difference in respect to demographic and anamnestic data.

The graduation of ureteral colic was from light, moderately severe, to extreme. Light and moderate ureteral colics were mostly found in the trial groups for Nitrolingual® forte capsules and butylscopolaminbromide, while severe ureteral colics were in excess in the trial groups for Nitrolingual®-Spray and Nitro Pohl® infus. Three extremely severe colics, who were not present in the other groups, were also found in this group.

The dosage for Nitrolingual® forte capsules was 1×2 capsules of 1.2 mg nitroglycerin; for Nitrolingual®-Spray 1×6 sprays per 0.4 mg nitroglycerin; for Nitro Pohl® infus 1×2, 2.4 mg nitroglycerin at 4 ml; and 1×1 20 mg butylscopolaminbromide in a 1 ml ampule. The intravenous administration of 2.4 mg nitroglycerin occurred over a time period of at least 5 minutes.

The evaluation parameters used to judge the success of the treatment 30 minutes after administration were good, moderate, and ineffective. To be classified as good, the success of the treatment had to provide a complete relief of pain. If residual pain existed the treatment was classified as a moderate success, and if a treatment with other medication was required within 30 minutes after application the treatment was labelled ineffective.

Beyond that, the recurrence frequency within the first 24 hours after application, the vital parameters, systolic and diastolic blood pressure, the pulse frequency, and the body temperature were included, as well as all undesirable drug effects.

Results

There were only slight differences observed between the trial groups in respect to relief of pain, with the statistical total remaining insignificant (fig. 1). A good to moderate pain relief was registered in 85% of the cases with Nitrolingual® forte, in 80% with Nitrolingual®-Spray, in 95% with Nitro Pohl® infus, and in 89.5% with butylscopolaminbromide, where a relatively high share of the patients (63%) were registered with only moderate pain relief. The difference between the groups, in terms of pain relief, remained statistically insignificant for slight, moderate, as well as for severe/extreme colics. The best results were achieved with Nitro Pohl® infus, especially in consideration of the fact that the group contained 3 extremely severe colics.

There were also not significant differences in the use of further therapeutic measures for residual pain within 30 minutes after application. In 30% of the cases, further analgesics and spasmolytics were used with Nitrolingual® forte. For Nitrolingual®-Spray, Nitro Pohl® infus, and for butylscopolaminbromide the further therapy measures amounted to 35, 30 and 47%, respectively. For slight to moderate colics there existed no difference in respect to the need for further therapeutic measures. There were noticeable statistical differences with severe to extreme colics. A further medication was necessary in all cases with Nitrolingual® capsules and butylscopolaminbromide.

There were no significant differences in the recurrence of ureteral colics within 24 hours after administration. They were observed with Nitrolingual® forte capsules and Nitro Pohl® infus in 42% of the cases, with Nitrolingual®-Spray in 25%, and with butylscopolaminbromide in 26% of the cases.

Among the Nitro groups there existed only slight, statistically insignificant, differences with respect to blood pressure levels.

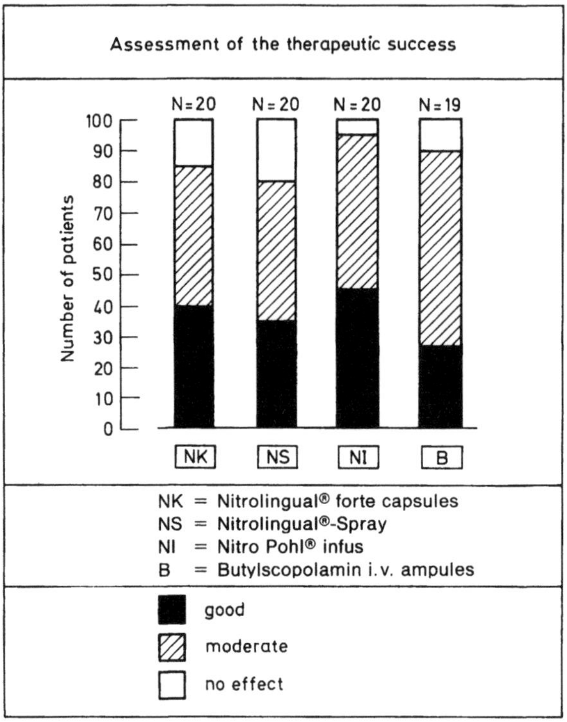

Fig. 1

The maximum systolic blood pressure decrease in the first half hour amounted for both Nitrolingual® forte capsules and spray to about 21 mmHg, for Nitro Pohl® infus 29.5 mmHg, and for butylscopolaminbromide 9.7 mmHg. The differences for all the nitroglycerin groups were significant compared with butylscopolaminbromide. The maximum diastolic blood pressure decrease within the first half hour after administration was also statistically significant in the nitroglycerin groups as compared with the butylscopolaminbromide group (9–12 mmHg maximum diastolic blood pressure decrease for the nitroglycerin groups versus 4.5 mmHg for the butylscopolaminbromide group.) Fig. 2 shows the mean change of the circulatory parameters at 10, 20, and 30 minutes after the application of the trial substance.

The pulse frequency increased slightly in all four groups, the differences remaining unremarkable. There were also no remarkable differences in reference to the laboratory parameters between the trial groups. A decrease of leucocytes and

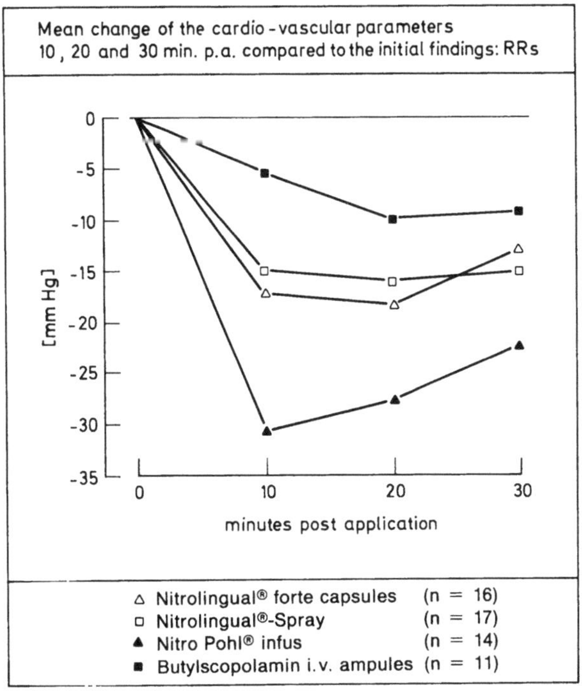

Fig. 2

creatinine was registered in the total collective, which can be explained as a result of the further nephrolithiasis treatment.

Differences in the frequency of undesirable drug effects were statistically noticeable. With Nitrolingual® forte capsules they were found in 15% of the cases, with Nitrolingual®-Spray in 40%, with Nitro Pohl® infus in 25%, and with butylscopolaminbromide in 5.3%.

The most frequent side-effects were observed with parenteral application (tab. 1). In one case the drop of systolic blood pressure below 80 mmHg had to be classified as intolerable. With the application of Nitrolingual®-Spray, headaches, dizziness, and sensation of heat were predominant. Taking multiple responses into consideration, it was observed ten times in total. In contrast, there were only three episodes of dizziness with the application of Nitrolingual® forte capsules. Therefore, with respect to undesirable drug effects Nitrolingual® forte capsules are preferable.

Table 1 Secondary effects

Symptoms	Nitrolingual® forte capsules	Nitrolingual®-Spray	Nitro Pohl® infus	Butylscopol-aminbromide
Dizziness	3	3	5	.
Headaches	.	4	.	.
Hypotonia	.	1	2	.
Nausea	.	.	2	1
Vomiting	.	.	2	.
Sensation of heat, flushing	.	2	.	.
Tingling	.	.	1	.

Discussion

Nitroglycerin has been a successful spasmolytic in the treatment of coronary disease for years. The intracellular point of attack for nitroglycerin is, after being transformed into a nitrosothiol, the calcium concentration. By accelerating the discharge into the extracellular space the intracellular concentration sinks, allowing a relaxation of the non-striated musculature. This spasmolytic acts not only on the vascular system, but also on the non-striated musculature of the ureter and can lead there to a pronounced pressure reduction of the ureter wall. Ultimately, this leads to a reduction of pain symptoms mediated by the extension receptors [2].

Therefore, a clinical trial of glycerol trinitrate for colics of the upper urinary tract was justifiable, especially if a randomized comparison were made with standard treatments. A further rationale for this clinical trial comes from the disputed use of combination preparations containing metamizole that, even though in very rare cases, may be connected with lethal complications.

A goal of this study was to make clear how far nitroglycerin and its efficacy could be compared to a standard treatment. Nitroglycerin, in all three different administration forms (Nitrolingual® forte capsules, Nitrolingual®-Spray, Nitro Pohl® infus), has proven itself as effective in clinical use as butylscopolaminbromide.

In over 90% a moderate or good pain relief was possible. In initial therapy with butylscopalaminbromide 26% obtained a complete relief of pain, whereas with glycerol trinitrate the levels ranged from 35 to 45%.

A moderate therapy effect was registered between 45 and 50% of the cases in the nitroglycerin groups, compared with 62.3% in the butylscopolamin group. In the nitroglycerin groups between 30 and 50% with moderate effects required further treatment. In the butylscopolaminbromide treated patients this was required in nearly all cases.

Remarkable is the relatively small portion of patients in the butylscopolaminbromide group who were fully free of pain as well as the relatively high portion of patients with partial therapy success. This means that in over half the patients an adjuvant therapy was necessary.

Among the individual kinds of administration with glycerol trinitrate there was no statistically significant difference shown with respect to the efficacy of initial pain relief, residual pain, additional therapeutic measures, and frequency of recurrence. Considering, however, the composition of the Nitro Pohl® infus group, where predominantly severe to extreme colics were found, it can be assumed that the intravenous administration of nitroglycerin is superior. That the frequency of undesirable drug effects in the nitroglycerin trial groups differed statistically was remarkable, compared with the butylscopolaminbromide control group, but was tolerable with the exception of a case of hypotonia.

Glycerol trinitrate has proven itself in a randomized comparison to standard treatments as an effective treatment for colics of the upper urinary tract. 2.4 mg of nitroglycerin is equivalent in terms of pain relief to 20 mg butylscopolamin. Based on the only slightly higher rate of undesirable drug effects on Nitrolingual® forte capsules when compared with the butylscopolaminbromide group, we would give preference to this application form.

Therapy with glycerol trinitrate represents, in our opinion, an improvement of the therapeutic treatment possibilities for ureteral colics. Future clinical studies should direct their attention mainly to the combination of glycerol trinitrate with other substances that are appropriate to extend the efficacy and durability of the spasmolysis. If necessary, a combination with a centrally effective analgesic would be of interest in the initial treatment of a ureteral colic. The abovementioned combination could allow a reduction of the relatively high concentration of glycerol trinitrate (2.4 mg).

References

[1] BGA-Mitteilung vom 27. 04. 1987 über das Ruhen der Zulassung von Kombinationspräparaten aus Metamizol und Spasmolytika bis zum 31. 12. 1988. Pharmazeutische Zeitung 132 (1987) Nr. 18.

[2] Dunzendorfer, U.: Zur Frage der Harnleiterspasmolyse durch Glyceroltrinitrate. In: H. Roskamm (Hrsg.): Nitroglycerin VI, Walter de Gruyter, Berlin – New York 1989.
[3] Kowalski, M.: Nitroglycerin bei Gallenkolik und spastischen Schmerzen der Gallenwege. Ärztl. Praxis *16* (1964) 1759.
[4] Sorkin, E. M., R. N. Brogden, I. A. Romankiewicz: Interavenous glyceroltrinitrate (nitroglycerin). A review of its pharmacological properties and therapeutic efficancy. Drugs *27* (1984) 45.

Glycerol trinitrate (sublingualspray) as a spasmolytic in biliary colics – first clinical experience

M. Staritz

Introduction

Biliary tract colic is the most frequent clinically severe, and, for the patient, painful symptom of cholecystolithiases. As cholecystolithiasis, which occurs in approximately 2.7 million gallstone carriers in West Germany, numbers among the most frequently occurring illnesses, it is assumed that approximately 1 million patients per year are affected by a colic.

For years, only one potent, established spasmolytic (butylscopolaminbromide) has been available for the treatment of this occurrence, one which is generally not dangerous but nevertheless highly painful for the patient. As the substance is not, for all practical purposes, enterally absorbed, administration in the form of a tablet or suppository is hardly effective. In the case of a biliary colic, its intravenous administration is therefore unavoidable. It follows that only a doctor can relieve the pain of a colic.

The identification of a spasmolytically effective, self-administrable substance, not requiring injection, would therefore be of great clinical significance.

Earlier studies were able to show that glycerol trinitrate has a strong relaxing effect on smooth musculature. This applies not only to the smooth musculature of the vascular system, for which reason the substance has been established as a primary medication for patients with coronary disease, arterial hypertension and pneumoedema, but also for the smooth musculature of the gastrointestinal tract. It could be shown that glycerol trinitrate has a relaxing effect on the smooth musculature of the biliary tract system.

A further advantage of the substance is that its full efficacy is reached within approximately one minute after sublingual application [1]. Ease of control of the substance, whose known potential side effects are headache and circulatory hypotension, is guaranteed by the first-pass mechanism of the substance through the liver, which results in the fact that the clinical concentration of a one-time sublingual application wears off within a half-life period of 5 minutes [1].

The goal of the pilot study was to find out whether a self-administered sublingual application of glycerol trinitrate is able to subdue colic pains in cholecystolithiasis. A dosage was selected which predicted adequate efficacy, but which, according to previous findings, precluded significant systemic side-effects.

In order to reach conditions as standardized as possible, only such patients were included in the testing procedure who had undergone extracorporeal shock wave lithotripsy under standardized conditions, and who exhibited a gallbladder concrement in crushed residual fragments with a defined diameter of 1–6 mm.

Method

18 patients who had undergone an extracorporeal shock wave lithotripsy (Siemens Lithostar plus, Siemens, Erlangen, FRG) under standardized conditions on gallbladder stones, were included in the study. The patient group was defined (table 1) on the basis of number of gallstones (n = 1, diameter 1–3 cm), the proven contractility of the gallbladder, and the sonographically measured disintegration success of the concrements. Gallbladder contractility was measured through sonographic determination of the gallbladder volume both before and 45 minutes after the administration of a standardized gastric stimulant, before the extracorporeal shock wave lithotripsy was carried out. The disintegration effect on solitary gallbladder stones was defined so that after one, to a maximum of three, lithotripsy sessions, residual fragments with a diameter not exceeding 6 mm were able to be sonographically detected in the gallbladder. It was discussed with the patients whether, should a colic appear, which occurs in over 30% of impulse lithotripsy treated patients, self-medication of glycerol trinitrate (Nitrolingual®-Spray, Pohl-Boskamp, Hohenlockstedt, FRG) should follow [2].

Treatment consisted of 3 consecutive applications of an 0.4 mg dosage of glycerol trinitrate spray to the tongue. In case no relief of pain was noted within approximately the first 5 minutes, medication was repeated once. In the total absence of therapeutical success, butylscopolaminbromide could then be administered by the family doctor or emergency doctor.

Table 1 Examined patients (n = 18)

- Condition after ESWL
- Female (age 23–64 years)
- unimpaired contractility of the gallbladder
- Diameter of the gallstone fragments of 1–6 mm

Results

A total of 21 cases of colics were noted during the observation period. Medication with Nitrolingual®-Spray led to a sharp decrease in symptoms in 19 of the 21 cases (90%). A repetition of the sublingual application was necessary in 6 of 21 cases (30%). In 3 cases, no relief of symptoms was achieved. In 6 of 21 cases, renewed painful symptoms of colic reappeared within a period of one hour (fig. 1).

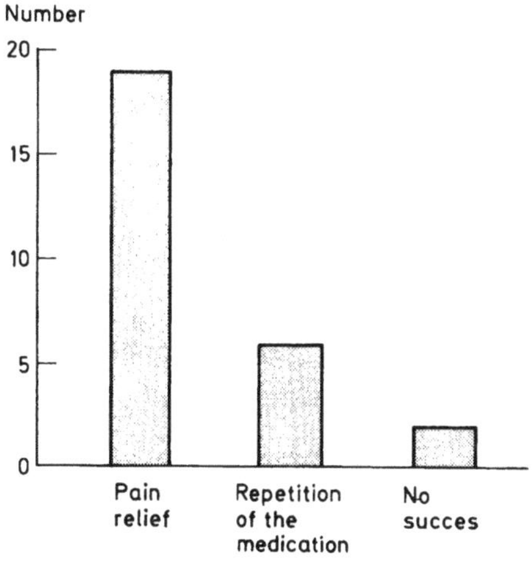

Fig. 1 Results in 21 colic cases.

Side effects

Serious clinical complications were not observed in any of the cases. In 20 of 21 applications, development of headache was noted after the administration of glycerol trinitrate. In 2 cases, circulatory hypotension was observed.

Discussion

The results of the first clinical studies of the use of glycerol trinitrate in gallstone colic show that the sublingual application of glycerol trinitrate (sublingual spray), represents an effective medication with few complications in the treatment of gallstone colic. A positive response to the treatment can be expected in up to 90% of the patients, and an increase in dosage is necessary in about one-third of the patients.

As the findings result from a study on only a limited number of cases, they must, of course, be interpreted with caution. A further limitation is that the symptom of "colic" was patient-defined, and the success of treatment was likewise measured by the patient, and not classified according to a pain-scoring system. On the other hand, it can be assumed that the well-informed patient is well-able to judge the symptoms of colic and, without the use of a pain-scale, subjectively decide whether the proffered medication leads to an improvement in the complaints.

A further limitation in this report of findings can be attributed to the lack of a placebo-treated control group. An administration of an ineffective placebo-medication was denied for ethical reasons. A comparison with an established-medication (butylscopolaminbromide), which requires intravenous administration, seemed to be more applicable.

The application of glycerol trinitrate provides the patient at all times with an immediately self-administrable medication – without serious side-effects, although cephalgia, a clinically insignificant side effect, must be accepted as almost obligatory. The duration of action of the substance is sufficient to hinder further colic symptoms in approximately 2/3 of the patients. It must be assumed that, because glycerol trinitrate has a half-life period of only 5 minutes, an application of the substance leads to lysis of spasms of the gallbladder. Considering the potential pressure-lowering effect of the substance, the number of patients tending towards a development of circulatory hypotension is relatively small. It should here be taken into account that, because of the pain, most patients prefer a reclining position, in which moderate circulatory hypotension is seldom noticed. Experiences gathered up to this point open up new possibilities. An expansion of previous findings in the form of a controlled study on a larger number of patients, should ensure the efficacy of the medication and enable an ideal dosage to be found. A further goal is to clarify whether further treatment, with an application of nitrate in retard form, is able to hinder a return of symptoms, or whether an application of analgetics if preferable. Finally, it appears to be necessary to find out whether the appearance of gallstone colic in up to 30% of gallstone carriers treated with an impulse lithotripsy, can be avoided through a consistent prophylactic application of nitrate.

References

[1] Armstrong, P. W., J. A. Armstrong, G. S. Marks: Blood levels after sublingual nitroglycerin. Circulation *59* (1979) 585–588.

[2] Sackmann, M., M. Delius, T. Sauerbruch et al.: Shock wave lithotripsy of gallbladder stones. The first 175 patients. N. Engl. J. Med. *318* (1988).

[4] Staritz, M., T. Poralla, K. Ewe et al.: Effect of glyceryl trinitrate on the sphincter of Oddi motility and baseline pressure. Gut. *26* (1985) 194–197.

[3] Staritz, M.: Pharmacology of the sphincter of Oddi. Endoscopy *20* (1988) 171–174.

Cardiac transplantation in Germany

R. Hetzer, M. Loebe, H. Warnecke, S. Schüler

Heart transplantation has become widely accepted as a safe and reliable treatment for irreversible heart failure, untreatable by any other medical or surgical means. Thus, more than 10 000 patients have been transplanted worldwide (fig. 1). The first heart transplantation in Germany was performed in 1969 in Munich, but, like in most other countries, this attempt was a failure. Heart transplantation was reintroduced in Germany, only after the introduction of cyclosporine, starting in Munich in 1981, followed by Hannover and Hamburg in 1983. Based on the experience of the Stanford Group under Shumway with rigid criteria for patient selection and improved postoperative monitoring, excellent results were obtained. In the International Registry for heart transplantation, the one-year survival rate now is 80%, and after 5 years, 74% of the heart transplant recipients are still alive (fig. 2). Aside from a very small number of heterotopic heart transplantations, it is mostly the technique of orthotopic heart transplantation as introduced by Shumway and Lower and modified by Cooley which is applied (fig. 3 a, b).

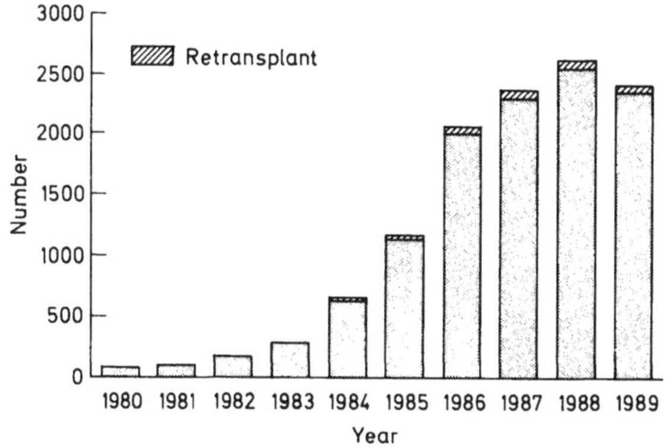

Fig. 1 Number of orthotopic heart transplants per year. Registry Int. Soc.for Heart Transplantation. J. Heart. Transplant. *9* (1990) 323.

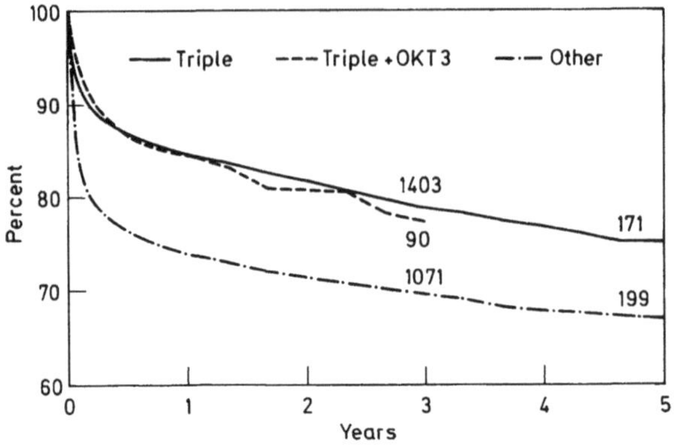

Fig. 2 Actuarial survival associated with heart transplantation by type of immunosuppression. J. Heart. Transpl. *9* (1990) 323. Tripple: Steroids, Acathioprin, Cyclosporin A.

Our own experience is based on 483 heart transplantations since 1983. The program was initiated at the Hannover Medical School (72 patients) and has been continued at the German Heart Center in Berlin since October 1985. The age of our recipients ranged between 3 months and 68 years, with a mean of 42.5 years. Indication for transplantation was dilated cardiomyopathy in 66% of all patients and coronary heart disease in 30% (see tab. 1). Seventy-eight patients had between one and four previous cardiac operations. Indication was congestive heart failure of class III and IV New York Heart Association in all patients, and four patients had had repeated resuscitation for intractible ventricular arrhythmias. Donor organs were negotiated almost exclusively through the Eurotransplant Organization, and some, most recently, were procured in the former GDR. Due to the large proportion of recipients dying while awaiting transplantation, donor acceptance has been greatly liberalized, particularly with older donors. The donor age ranged from 12 months to 55 years with a mean of 37.8 years. Comparative studies with respect to donor age have shown no significant difference in the immediate and late performance of the hearts. All patients received triple immunosuppressive therapy, consisting of azathioprine, cyclosporin A, and steroids. Over the years, the basic immunosuppressive regimen has been modified 4 times. Recently patients received cyclosporin A, 4 mg/kg body weight, immediately before transplantation. This is increased to whole blood levels of 600 to 800 ng/ml and then lowered to 400/500 ng/ml in the chronic phase beyond 3 months after transplantation. An increasing number of patients are now taken off chronic steroid medication, particularly children,

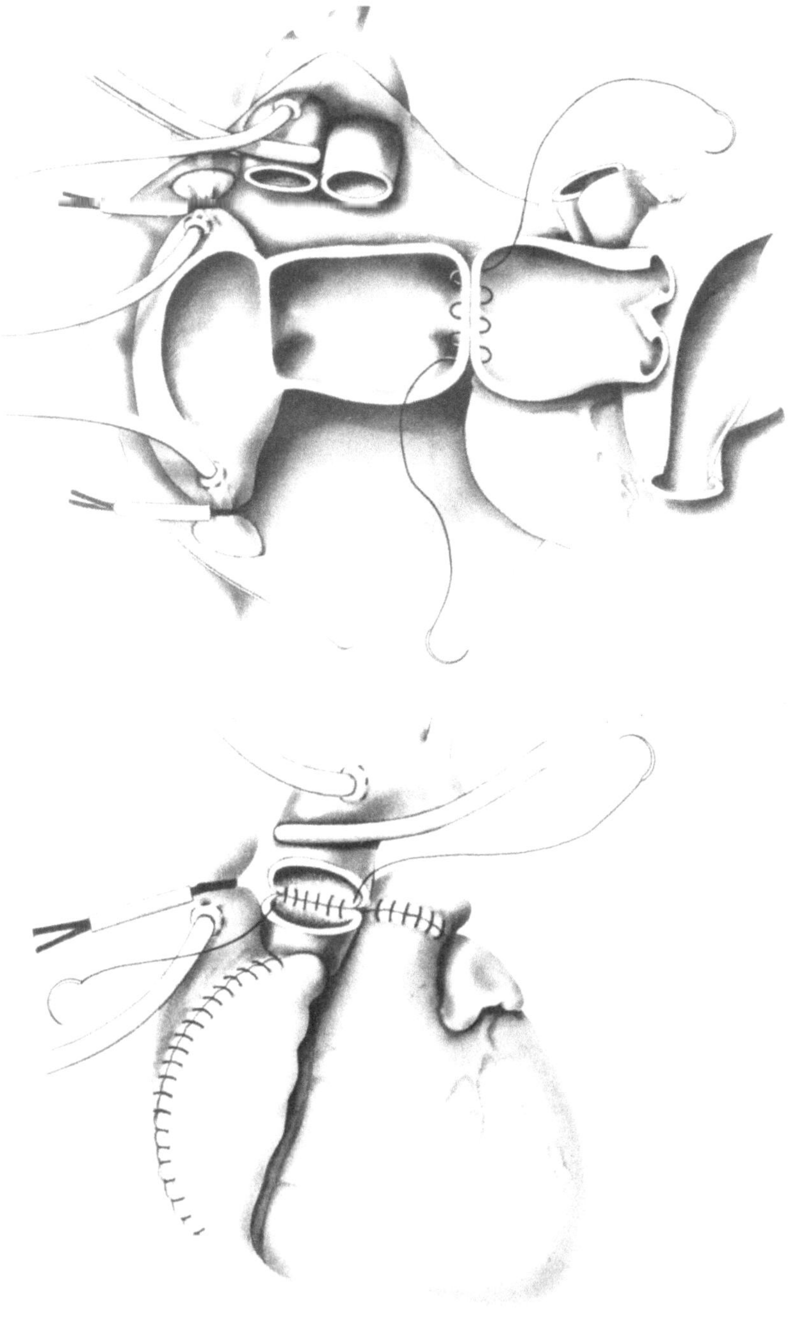

Fig. 3 Operative technique in orthotopic heart transplantation
a) Implantation beginning at the left atrium
b) Completion of implantation

Table 1 Preoperative diagnosis (483 patients)

	Number of patients
Congestive cardiomyopathy	320
Coronary artery disease	144
– Previous operation	78
Mitral valve replacement	6
Aortic valve replacement	6
Endocardial fibrosis	4
Tricuspid atresia	1
Right ventricular dysplasia	1
Hypoplastic left heart syndrome	1

patients older than 55, and all those with insulin-dependent diabetes and signs of osteoporosis. Rejection monitoring has relied on repeated endomyocardial biopsy. Within our group, we developed the technique of monitoring the patient via an intramyocardial electrogram which has allowed day by day monitoring during the patient's sleeping phase and via distant monitoring through the telephone system. M-mode echocardiography and cytoimmunologic monitoring have been quite helpful but were not able to substitute invasive monitoring. All patients were examined by ventriculography and coronary angiography at 3 months and then yearly after transplantation. Over a 5 year period, hemodynamics remained remarkably stable with a slight trend to hypertension, afterload increase, and some left ventricular decrease of ejection fraction. While in the early postoperative course right heart failure due to increased pulmonary vascular resistance of the recipient was responsible for graft failure, in the long term course this was due to accelerated arterial sclerosis in the transplanted heart (tab. 2). Coronary artery disease was observed in 30 patients. In an analysis of those patients who developed coronary artery disease after transplantation, we discovered cytomegalovirus infection as a major risk factor. The incidence of CMV infection in this group was 66%, as compared to 35% in patients who did not develop coronary artery disease.

Physical and psychological rehabilitation has been very successful in the surviving patients. 40% returned to work, school, or normal household activities, 39% are leading an active retirement, and 21% are planning return to work.

As a large proportion of recipients died before reaching transplantation, we initiated a program of mechanical bridging to transplant at our institution in July of 1987. We used both the total artificial heart and the mechanical assist

Table 2 Causes of death (142 patients)

	Number of patients
Rejection	29
Infection	62
Graft failure	30
– Acute, biventricular	14
– Acute, right ventricular	10
– Chronic, CAD	6
Cerebral complications	4
Others	17

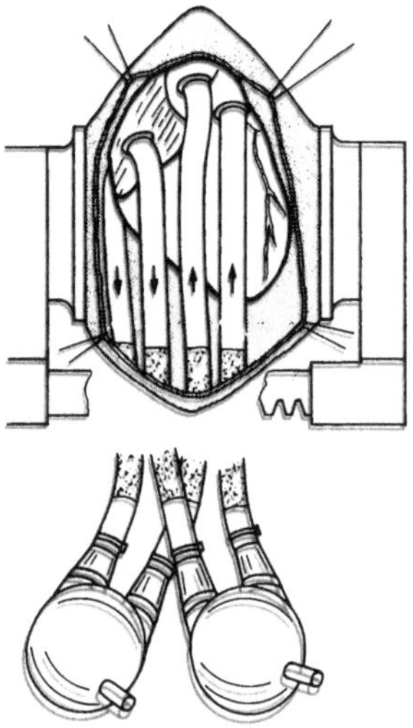

Fig. 4 Biventricular assist device. Cannulation: right atrium, pulmonary artery as right ventricular bypass and left atrium aorta as left ventricular bypass.

devices designed and constructed by the team of Bücherl, Berlin (fig. 4, 5). Till now, 31 patients have undergone mechanical bridging periods of a few hours to 53 days. Of these patients, 13 died on the bridging system from further deterioration and development of sepsis. Heart transplantations were successfully carried out in 18 patients. The survival in this group of patients is comparable to that in the patients following primary transplantation.

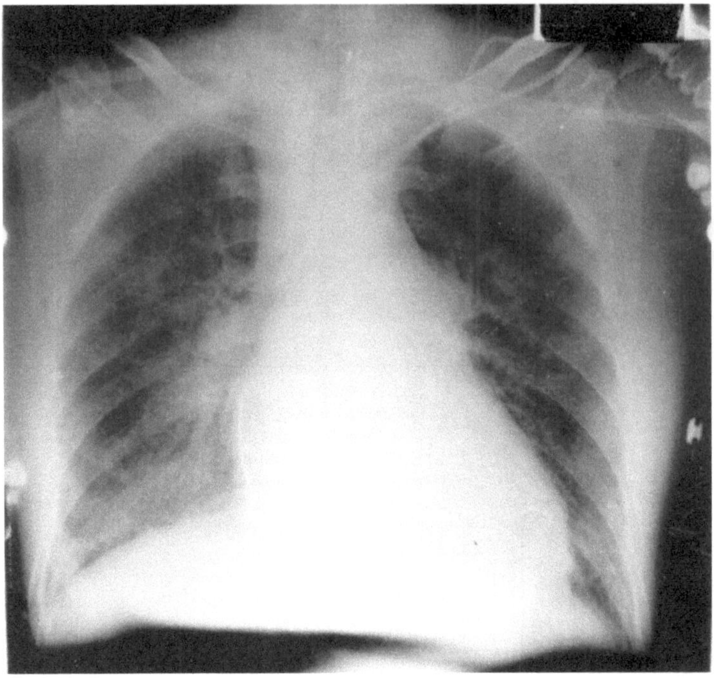

Fig. 5 Thorax X-ray after implantation of biventricular assist device.

Heart transplantation has become an accepted treatment for patients with irreversible heart failure. The major limiting factor for this type of treatment is still the insufficient number of available donor hearts. Therefore, the development of alternative types of treatment, such as permanent mechanical support or xenogenic transplantation, remains a major challenge.

Multicentre trials in acute myocardial infarction in Canada and the US: myocardial salvage and remodelling

B. I. Jugdutt

Introduction

Acute myocardial infarction (AMI) remains a major cause of death and disability world-wide. The Killip classification [19] of patients with AMI and expected mortality in the 1970's is well known. Advances in coronary care and post-AMI management since then have improved the mortality figures somewhat, as reflected in data from Cairns and colleagues [1]. Nevertheless, early survivors are at risk for ventricular aneurysm formation and congestive heart failure. In 1978, Hutchins and Bulkley [5] recognized that early infarct expansion without new necrosis is a major cause of morbidity and mortality of AMI. In 1979, Eaton et al. [2] first reported the recognition of regional left ventricular dilatation or infarct expansion from serial imaging with two-dimensional echocardiography (2D-echo) over the first 2 weeks after AMI in 28 patients. It became clear in the 1980's that complications after AMI are related not only to the total infarct size, but also to the severity of left ventricular remodelling or topographic deterioration and left ventricular dilatation that take place during healing and in turn adversely affect left ventricular function and outcome.

Our studies since 1980, and those from other laboratories, indicate that healing after AMI is progressive and is associated with progressive remodelling. The time scale is for dogs and should be extended for humans.

At the histopathologic and biochemical levels there is a sequence of acute inflammation, chronic inflammation and necrosis when the infarct is relatively "soft", followed by fibroblast proliferation and collagen deposition which cements the early deformation and results in a firm scar.

At the structural level there is early remodelling with early regional expansion, with stretching, some thinning and dilatation. Later there is collagen compaction, more marked thinning and increased distensibility.

At the molecular level there is an acute decrease in the number of myocytes across the wall with expansion. Later collagen fibrils establish connections with live myocytes and resist distension. Nevertheless, progressive dilatation occurs, especially with large transmural infarcts, leading to left ventricular (LV) aneurysm, LV volume overload, LV hypertrophy and congestive heart failure.

Major factors involved in remodelling include infarct size, transmurality, adequacy of healing and mechanical deformation forces, especially preload, afterload and wall stress [20, 21].

Results from our laboratory and others indicate that therapy to limit remodelling should be targeted at both early and late phases of therapy. The potential to limit remodelling and improve or preserve function is greater with therapy in the early phase.

We have shown, experimentally, that low dose intravenous nitroglycerin therapy over 6 hours after acute myocardial infarction reduces pathologic infarct size relative to the region at risk [11] in a conscious dog model. The beneficial effects were associated with reduced preload and afterload, and increased collateral blood flow. Such short-term therapy also reduced infarct expansion or remodelling measured 7 days later [8]. In the same model when nitroglycerin-induced hypotension was excessive down to mean arterial pressures below 80 mmHg, coronary perfusion was impaired, collateral flow did not increase and infarct size was not reduced [7]. In fact, infarct size was increased with marked nitroglycerin-induced hypotension, emphasizing the need for cautious titration of dose to a safe level.

In the rat model, Pfeffer et al. [3, 25] demonstrated progressive left ventricular dilatation and its relation to mortality and morbidity. Pfeffer's group [24, 26, 27] later showed attenuation of left ventricular dilatation, improved left ventricular function and decreased survival with chronic captopril therapy. In the dog model, we showed that chronic isosorbide dinitrate therapy during healing after AMI improves left ventricular geometry, and decreases left ventricular distensibility [9]. Later we showed that chronic isosorbide dinitrate, captopril and enalapril therapy improve left ventricular geometry and function in the same model [10, 12, 13].

From this background it is clear that the scope of myocardial salvage should be expanded to include salvage of ventricular muscle as well as ventricular geometry and function. New therapeutic strategies should consider all possible ways of preserving muscle, geometry and function from the time of onset of acute myocardial infarction to the completion of the healing process over six weeks or more.

Pathophysiologic studies indicate that the early hours after AMI are pivotal in our efforts to limit myocardial necrosis, remodelling and ventricular dysfunction.

Short-term nitroglycerin therapy

In 1988 we published the final results of a large randomized, placebo-controlled, single-blinded clinical trial of low dose intravenous nitroglycerin therapy for the first forty-eight hours after acute myocardial infarction [17]. There were 310 patients; 154 patients received nitroglycerin therapy and 156 patients were placebo controls, who received 5% dextrose in water at a constant rate of 1 ml/min. for 48 hours. The treated group received low dose nitroglycerin therapy to decrease mean blood pressure by 10% in normotensives and by 30% in hypertensives. This method of administration was based on our experimental data and clinical data from other groups (including Bussmann, Flaherty and Jaffe), whose data we have summarized [15].

The results indicated that low dose nitroglycerin infusion in AMI was safe, limited infarct size and infarct expansion, decreased major infarct-related complications and improved in-hospital and one-year survival. Myocardial salvage, assessed by cumulative creatine kinase infarct size, was demonstrated with both anterior and interior infarct locations and with early or late timing of therapy. However, salvage was greatest with early therapy, within 4 hours of symptoms. Further, salvage was still evident with therapy within 10 hours of onset of AMI. Myocardial salvage was also greater in the subgroup with mean arterial pressure above 80 mmHg. Regional left ventricular dysfunction or asynergy decreased, and left ventricular ejection fraction improved with nitroglycerin. Infarct expansion and thinning were less with nitroglycerin. Functional class improved with nitroglycerin. Other major infarct-related complications were also less with nitroglycerin including the clinical infarct expansion syndrome, infarct extension, heart block, left ventricular thrombus, cardiogenic shock and in-hospital mortality. More important, nitroglycerin decreased mortality up to one year but this effect was mainly in the anterior transmural or Q-wave infarction subgroup.

Hemodynamic tolerance during low dose intravenous nitroglycerin therapy in that study developed in less than 25% of patients [18]. It blunted the beneficial effect on infarct size but positive effects on function, topography and complications persisted. Thus, tolerance should not deter the use of low dose nitroglycerin therapy in AMI. Yusuf et al. [30] recently performed meta analysis of pooled data from individual clinical trials in North America and Europe using intravenous nitrates in AMI and found a highly significant 35% reduction in the odds of death.

Prolonged nitrate therapy

The next question was whether therapy during the later phase of healing after AMI can produce additional benefit. Thus, experimentally, oral nitroglycerin therapy during the first week after anterior AMI improved left ventricular function, mechanical strength, resistance to distension and presumably reduced aneurysm formation at 6 weeks in the dog model in our laboratory [9]. Recently we reported that prolonged nitroglycerin therapy, given intravenously for the first 48 hours followed by buccal nitrate for 6 weeks (t.i.d., allowing an 8-hour nitrate free interval to avoid tolerance) after anterior Q-wave AMI in patients at our hospital, resulted in long-term preservation of left ventricular topography and improvement of left ventricular function in a randomized, placebo-controlled, double-blind study of 56 patients [22]. The benefit persisted for up to 8.5 months after discontinuation of therapy [14].

Potential mechanisms

The mechanisms for benefit with nitroglycerin include: improved hemodynamics (decreased preload, afterload and wall stress), improved cardiac geometry, improved flow and perfusion, improved regional and global performance, decreased infarct size and decreased infarct related complications.

Other therapies

Limitation of infarct remodelling can be achieved by diverse therapeutic interventions via diverse mechanisms. The angiotensin-converting-enzyme (ACE) inhibitors, captopril and enalapril have also been shown to be powerful agents for reducing remodelling after AMI in our dog model [13].

Thrombolytic therapy, which restores antegrade coronary flow and salvages muscle, has been shown to improve survival in both the large Italian GISSI trial [4] and the international ISIS-2 trial [6].

Although successful coronary reperfusion is associated with salvage of geometry, it does not always result in prompt salvage of function. This dissociation between salvage of geometry and function might be due to myocardial stunning and reperfusion injury. However, adjunctive therapy can be used for prompt recruitment of ventricular function in that setting, as we have shown with intravenous nitroglycerin [29]. The effect of intravenous nitroglycerin and late reperfusion with angioplasty and streptokinase was studied in a randomized trial of 73 patients. The results on left ventricular ejection fraction are shown and indicate prompt recovery in the nitroglycerin groups. Multicenter trials currently still in progress, using prolonged therapy with ACE inhibitors such as captopril (SAVE study) or enalapril (SOLVD study) after AMI, are targeted mainly on the later phase of remodelling after AMI. Recently, Sharpe et al. [28] found that chronic captopril therapy one week after Q-wave AMI limited left ventricular dilatation and improved left ventricular ejection fraction after one month and up to one year in a randomized double-blind study of 60 patients (captopril; furosemide; placebo). Also, Pfeffer et al. [23] showed that chronic captopril therapy after 11 to 31 day old anterior Q-wave AMI limited left ventricular dilatation and improved exercise capacity during one year follow-up in a randomized, double-blind placebo controlled study of 59 patients (captopril 30; placebo 29).

Our own trial compares prolonged therapy with captopril and nitrate throughout the healing phase after AMI.

Prolonged nitrate versus prolonged nitrate plus captopril

We recently reported [16] preliminary data from a randomized, double-blind, placebo-controlled study which was begun in 1988. Briefly, we posed the following questions:

1. What is the long term impact of chronic therapy with nitroglycerin or captopril, or both, between 48 hours and 6 weeks after acute transmural (Q-wave) myocardial infarction on LV geometry and function?
2. Does the benefit seen at 6 weeks persist after therapy is discontinued?

We used a 2×2 factorial design (4 groups of patients).

Pre-randomization standard treatment consisted of:

Low dose intravenous nitroglycerin infusion for 48 hours.

- Dose titration to decrease mean blood pressure by 10% in normotensive and 30% in hypertensives
- but not below 80 mmHg.

Post-randomization treatment regimens consisted of a "double dummy" design with:

- Captopril: 6.25 – 12.5 mg t.i.d. oral; average dose 12.5 mg t.i.d.
- Nitrate: 1 – 3 mg t.i.d. buccal; average dose 2 mg t.i.d.

Eccentric dosing 5 hourly (08:00, 13:00, and 18:00 hours (with 8-hour "washout" period).

- For both, the initial dose was titrated over 2 days so that mean blood pressure did not fall by more than 10%.
- Placebo: matched placebo for captopril or nitrate regimen.

The preliminary data involved 80 patients with 20 per cell.

Left ventricular ejection fraction, by Simpson's rule, was unchanged with placebo but improved with active therapies and effect persisted up to 1 year after discontinuing therapy.

The beneficial effects included: decreased LV volumes, decreased LV asynergy, decreased expansion, decreased thinning, increased LV ejection fraction, decreased LV aneurysms, improved morbidity parameters. However, there was no difference in benefit after chronic therapy with captopril or nitrate or captopril plus nitrate.

In conclusion, our future attempts at myocardial salvage after AMI should be targeted at ventricular muscle, geometry and function throughout the healing process. Early intravenous nitroglycerin followed by either nitrate or an ACE-inhibitor or both might be the way of the future in the management of patients after AMI.

References

[1] Cairns, J. A., J. Singer, M. Gent et al.: One year mortality outcomes of all coronary and intensive care unit patients with acute myocardial infarction, unstable angina or other chest pain in Hamilton, Ontario, a city of 375,000 people. Can. J. Cardiol. *5* (1989) 239–246.

[2] Eaton, L. W., J. L. Weiss, B. H. Bulkley et al.: Regional cardiac dilatation after acute myocardial infarction: Recognition by two-dimensional echocardiography. N. Engl. J. Med. *300* (1979) 57–62.

[3] Fletcher, P. J., J. M. Pfeffer, M. A. Pfeffer et al.: Left ventricular diastolic pressure-volume relations in rats with healed myocardial infarction. Effects on systolic function. Circ. Res. *49* (1981) 618–626.

[4] Gruppo Italiano per lo Studio della Streptochinasi nell' Infarcto Miocardico. Long-term effects of intravenous thrombolysis in acute myocardial infarction: Final report of the GISSI study. Lancet *2* (1987) 871–874.

[5] Hutchins, G. M., B. H. Bulkley: Infarct expansion versus extension: Two different complications of acute myocardial infarction. Am. J. Cardiol. *41* (1978) 1127–1132.

[6] ISIS 2 (2nd International Study of Infarct Survival) Collaborative Group. Randomized trial of intravenous streptokinase, oral aspirin, both, or neither among 17, 187 cases of suspected acute myocardial infarction: ISIS 2. Lancet II (1988) 349–360.

[7] Jugdutt, B. I.: Myocardial salvage by intravenous nitroglycerin in conscious dogs: Loss of beneficial effect with marked nitroglycerin-induced hypotension. Circulation *68* (1983) 673–684.

[8] Jugdutt, B. I.: Delayed effects of early infarct-limiting therapies on healing after acute myocardial infarction. Circulation *72* (1985) 907–914.

[9] Jugdutt, B. I.: Effect of nitroglycerin and ibuprofen on left ventricular topography and rupture threshold during healing after myocardial infarction in the dog. Can. J. Physiol. Pharmacol. *66* (1988) 385–395.

[10] Jugdutt, B. I.: Improved left ventricular geometry and function during healing after anterior and interior infarction in the dog. (Abstr). Circulation *78* (Suppl. II) (1988) 643.

[11] Jugdutt, B. I., L. C. Becker, G. M. Hutchins et al.: Effect of intravenous nitroglycerin on collateral blood flow and infarct size in the conscious dog. Circulation *63* (1981) 17–28.

[12] Jugdutt, B. I., M. Ibrahim, J. Demare: Functional impact of remodelling therapy with captopril and nitroglycerin during healing after acute myocardial infarction. (Abstr). Clin. Invest. Med. *13* (1990) C44.

[13] Jugdutt, B. I., B. L. Michorowski, B. F. O'Kelly: Pharmacologic modification of left ventricular remodeling during healing after myocardial infarction. (Abstr). J. Am. Coll. Cardiol. *11* (1988) 252A.

[14] Jugdutt, B. I., B. L. Michorowski, W. J. Tymchak: Peristent improvement in left ventricular geometry and function after anterior transmural myocardial infarction by prolonged nitroglycerin therapy. (Abstr). Europ. Heart J. *11* (Suppl.) (1990) 190.

[15] Jugdutt, B. I., B. A. Sussex, W. J. Tymchak et al.: Intravenous nitroglycerin in the early management of acute myocardial infarction. Cardiovasc. Rev. Rep. *10* (1989) 29–35.

[16] Jugdutt, B. I., W. Tymchak, D. Humen et al.: Prolonged nitroglycerin versus captopril therapy on remodelling after transmural myocardial infarction. (Abstr). Circulation *82* (Suppl. III) (1990) 442.

[17] Jugdutt, B. I., J. W. Warnica: Intravenous nitroglycerin therapy to limit myocardial infarct size, expansion and complications: Effect of timing, dosage and infarct location. Circulation *78* (1988) 906–919.

[18] Jugdutt, B. I., J. W. Warnica: Tolerance with low dose intravenous nitroglycerin therapy in acute myocardial infarction. Amer. J. Cardiol. *64* (1989) 581–587.

[19] Killip, T., J. T. Kimball: Treatment of myocardial infarction in a coronary care unit. A two-year experience with 250 patients. Am. J. Cardiol. *20* (1967) 457–464.

[20] Michorowski, B. L., P. J. Senaratne, B. I. Jugdutt: Deterring Myocardial Infarct Expansion. Cardiovasc. Rev. Rep. *8* (1987) 55–62.

[21] Michorowski, B. L., P. J. Senaratne, B. I. Jugdutt: Myocardial Infarct Expansion. Cardiovasc. Rev. Rep. *8* (1987) 42–47.

[22] Michorowski, B. L., W. T. Tymchak, B. I. Jugdutt: Improved left ventricular function and topography by prolonged nitroglycerin therapy after acute myocardial infarction. (Abstr). Circulation *76* (Suppl. IV) (1987) 128.

[23] Pfeffer, M. A., G. A. Lamas, D. E. Vaughan et al.: Effect of captopril on progressive ventricular dilatation after anterior myocardial infarction. N. Engl. J. Med. *319* (1988) 80.

[24] Pfeffer, J. M., M. A. Pfeffer, E. Braunwald: Influence of chronic captopril therapy on the infarcted left ventricle of the rat. Circ. Res. *57* (1985) 84–95.

[25] Pfeffer, M. A., J. M. Pfeffer, M. C. Fishbein et al.: Myocardial infarct size and ventricular function in rats. Circ. Res. *44* (1979) 503–512.

[26] Pfeffer, M. A., J. M. Pfeffer, C. Steinberg et al.: Survival after experimental myocardial infarction: Beneficial effects of long-term therapy with captopril. Circulation *72* (1985) 406–412.

[27] Pfeffer, M. A., J. M. Pfeffer: Ventricular enlargement and reduced survival after myocardial infarction. Circulation *75* (Suppl. IV) (1987) 93–97.

[28] Sharpe, N., J. Murphy, H. Smith et al.: Treatment of patients with symptomless left ventricular dysfunction after myocardial infarction. Lancet *1* (1988) 255–259.

[29] Tymchak, W. J., B. L. Michorowski, J. R. Burton et al.: Preservation of left ventricular function and topography with combined reperfusion and intravenous nitroglycerin in acute myocardial infarction. (Abstr). J. Am. Coll. Cardiol. *11* (1988) 90A.

[30] Yusuf, S., R. Collins, S. MacMahon et al.: Effect of IV nitrates on mortality in acute myocardial infarction: An overview of randomized trials. Lancet *1* (1988) 1088–1092.

Treatment of patients with myocardial infarction in the USSR

E. I. Chazov

Traditionally Soviet physicians have paid great attention to the problems of myocardial infarction (MI) since the first clinical description of this disease in 1909 by Obraztsov and Strazhesko. In 1959 from on our observations made in the clinic headed by Professor A. L. Myasnikov, the basic principles of myocardial infarction treatment have been elaborated. These principles are still fundamental in the organization of MI treatment.

Though since then our knowledge about the mechanisms of MI development has enlarged considerably, including the details of formation of necrosis, foci and border zones, the typical features of arrhythmias, the development of heart failure etc. Two main principles remain still the most important:

1. The success of treatment to a large degree depends on the time interval between the onset of acute coronary insufficiency and the beginning of the required full-scale therapy. The fate of the patients with myocardial infarction and the prognosis of the disease depends on how fast the physicians having modern methods of diagnosis and treatment can reach the patient.
2. In a vast majority of cases, the real reason for the development of myocardial infarction is thrombosis of coronary vessels leading not only to necrosis but also to formation of peri-infarcted zones. Therefore, at present the methods of choice are thrombolytic therapy or mechanical destruction of thrombus.

In the western hemisphere these principles were described in particular in a book "Thrombosis and Embolics in Internal Diseases Treatment", published in West Germany in 1974.

The first principle was widely realized due to our system of ambulances. This system of ambulances is composed of the teams, central station and district stations. The team consists of one physician and one or two trained nurses who possess portable equipment for diagnostics and a set of drugs. The team may reach a patient within 15–20 min. at any place and begin to exert suitable medical help, either at home or during transportation of the patients to the hospital. Any citizen of our country dialing 03 in any city or country of the

USSR may call such team free of charge. This speed is achieved due to the fact that in addition to the central ambulance stations in large cities we have a highly developed network of so-called district stations, located in all regions of the city where the personnel on duty is located. For example in Moscow we have forty five district stations of this type.

What are the advantages of this system of ambulance teams? It is well known that the early therapy of the pain syndrome and arrhythmia is an important prerequisite of the prevention of some types of cardiogenic shock and sudden death. However, at present the main task of these teams as well as any physician treating MI patients is to ensure the earliest possible therapy by thrombolytics.

When we reported at the National Institute of Health in Bethesda (USA) in 1963 our data dealing with the first experience of thrombolytics in the myocardial infarction patients we could not think, taking into consideration the scepticism existing at that time, that the method would become a leading method of MI treatment. The treatment by thrombolytics is based on the fact that in the majority of cases the occlusion of coronary vessels is the main cause of the circulation disturbances in heart muscle leading to formation of the necrosis zone.

Since 1963 thrombolytic therapy has shown a great evolution. Thrombus dissolution depends on the activity of thrombolytic agents, their concentration in the zone of thrombus formation and the duration of its action. Taking into consideration these factors, we were seeking new thrombolytic agents and better methods of their administration. Of great importance is the reduction of possible side effects of these agents, e. g. toxicity, haemorraghic complications, allergic reactions, etc.

At present in clinical practice all over the world and in our country, in particular, clinicians use streptokinase (streptase), urokinase, tissue plasminogen activator (rt-PA) and other thrombolytics. Each of these agents possesses certain advantages and disadvantages. In addition to these agents we use a thrombolytic agent streptodecase created in the USSR. This is a form of streptokinase immobilized on dextran matrix.

The immobilization on the dextran allowed to decrease 30 times the antigenic properties of the drug, to reduce significantly toxic and allergic reactions of the streptokinase, and what is the most important, to prolong the term of thrombolytic activity after a single injection for up to 3 days.

An important step to extend the possibilities of thrombolytic therapy is the development of the method of intracoronary infusion of the thrombolytics. In 1975 we demonstrated for the first time the possibility of intracoronary infusion of thrombolytics. However, our experience demonstrated that the method is of limited practical value, because of the organizational problems and high cost due to the angiography, which is required to control the procedure.

At present another approach to the application of thrombolytics for the treatment of MI patients is actively used. The involvement of well-trained personnel, diagnostic and clinical facilities, the possibility to perform cardioversion in the ambulance allows us to begin thrombolytic therapy in the first hours of the disease at a prehospital stage, e. g. at home or during transportation. Any citizen of our country may use these possibilities free of charge.

What are the advantages of such an approach? This question will be answered by the comparative data of two groups of patients treated by thrombolytics.

The first group was treated according to a routine protocol. In other words, a patient was transported in an intensive care unit in a hospital, where coronary angiography was performed. If the results of the angiography indicated the existence of the occlusion then the patient is treated by thrombolytic therapy. In case of a success reperfusion occurs only after 5.5 hours.

For the second group of patients the infusion of thrombolytics was started at the prehospital stage right after the diagnosis was established. On average the beginning of the therapy was as quick as 1.4 hour after the angina attack. The patients of these two groups enter the hospital at the same time. However, at the time of hospitalization the infusion of thrombolytics to the patients of the second group was practically terminated. According to coronary angiography data, the reperfusion in these cases occurred within 3 hours after the beginning of attack.

The data of the first coronary angiography for the patients of the first group which hadn't received thrombolytics at the prehospital stage show that the occlusion of infarct-related artery was found in 88% of cases. At the same time in a group with an early prehospital thrombolysis occlusion was found in 15% of patients, whereas 85% of patients possessed patent arteries. In case of prehospital treatment we used intravenous infusion of streptokinase at the dosage of 1.000.000 units during 20 min.

Under conditions of early prehospital usage of thrombolytics we analyzed the development of two complications, i. e. life-threatening arrhythmias and haemorrhages. However, the frequency of these complications was equal for the both groups of patients. In no case did these complications lead to a lethal outcome. Heart failure was more rare in the group of out of hospital treated patients. These differences persisted in a long-term follow-up of the results, for example at one year after infarction. The mortality in this group at the end of the first year was 5%, being much lower than in a group of patients treated with later reperfusion (4–6 hours).

In addition to streptokinase, streptodecase and urokinase, we have carried out the analysis of the efficacy of several types of tissue plasminogen activators.

The drug was used within first 5 hours of the disease after angiographic verification of the infarct-related artery occlusion. An average time of the start of infusion was 4 hours after the beginning of the attack. We have used the following schedule: 10 mg were administered as a bolus injection with a subsequent infusion of the drug during 3 hours with a rate of 50 mg during the first hour and 20 mg during the following hours. A total dose was equal to 100 mg. During the first five days of the disease the patients were treated by intravenous infusion of heparin with a rate of 1.000 units per hour. After 90 min. after the beginning of plasminogen active infusion coronary reperfusion was found in 63% of cases, while in coronary angiography after 180 min. of reperfusion it reached 70% of patients.

In addition to a high efficacy of tissue plasminogen activator one should pay attention to high incidence (up to 20%) of rethrombosis in the course of such treatment.

The successful treatment of MI greatly depends on the efficacy of prevention and treatment of its complications especially during the first hours of the disease. First of all one should suppress the pain syndrome. Usually it disappears in the course of thrombolytic therapy. In the USSR we often use the inhalation of the mixture of NO with oxygen by a special small device. In case of a severe and prolonged pain syndrome we successfully use peridural anaesthesia with administration of 2% lidocain solution, 80 mg every 2 hours. From our observations we concluded that peridural anaesthesia does not possess a significant effect on such hemodynamic indices as mean arterial pressure, heart rate and ejection fraction.

A very threatening complication is arrhythmia, especially ventricular tachycardia and fibrillation. For the treatment of such complications we used for the first time the antiarrhythmic drug Etmozin synthesized in the USSR. The drug was especially effective in the treatment of ventricular extrasystoles. The drug produced now in USA is coming to American clinics. At present we have completed the clinical trials and switched to clinical application for the treatment of MI patients with arrhythmia a new drug. This is a plant alkaloid isolated from aconitum leicostomum.

When discussing the problems of MI treatment one cannot miss to look for of agents that may affect peri-infarction injury influencing its metabolism and restricting the area of MI. We have studied the effect of different drugs, e. g. hyaluronidase, verapamil, phosphocreatine, antioxidants and nitroglycerin. Nitroglycerin infusion was found to be the most efficient. We have studied its effect both in experimental test systems and in the clinic, where we use this agent for more than 15 years. This agent activates the enzymes involved in oxidation-reduction processes in cardiomyocytes (such as succinatedehydrogenase, lactatedehydrogenease, glucoso-6-phosphatedehydrogenase), protects nerve terminals and activates plastic processes. According to the data of pro cardiac mapping of ECG, the analysis of enzyme activity, necrosis markers, intravenous administration of nitroglycerin promotes the limitation of the foci of the lesion.

Using other therapeutic agents, we have observed fast positive dynamics of ST segment and the reduction of the frequency of cardiac failure development in a group of patients treated by phosphocreatine. At present a new antioxidant – hystochrome – created in the USSR is at the stage of clinical trials. We currently analyse the effect of this drug on myocardial infarction development.

This paper considers some of the basic approaches and problems of MI therapy. While these problems are much more numerous and their number is still increasing we are unable to discuss all of them because of lack of time. Among these problems I may just mention those, connected with coronary bypass surgery in threatening situations, the basic approaches to the treatment of cardiac failure, therapy by beta-blockers, CA-antagonists and acetylcysteine etc.

Although the search for new methods of treatment and new effective drugs is very arduous and hard it should be continued in spite of all difficulties. During the past 30 years we succeeded to reduce the hospital mortality in MI patients from 22% in 1959 to 8.5% in 1989. Such figures are not unique today. We consider that the success achieved in the therapy of MI patients is a result of the biomedical science all over the world. This result is achieved thanks to the unification of the scientists from different countries and we still have reserves in this field. We must continue this work keeping in mind the motto of the ancient clinicians: "Per aspera, ad astra", "Overcoming problems – to the stars". And this is worth doing, since the prize is so high, i. e. human life.

Case discussion

Moderator: P. G. Hugenholtz

Hugenholtz: We are dealing with a 73-year old patient with a long history of hypertension. In 1986 it deteriorated and cardiac insufficiency occurred. The patient was treated with aortic-coronary bypasses due to angina pectoris. The preoperative thoracic x-ray showed a clearly enlarged dilated heart. The ECGs did not further assist in the diagnosis. In any case there was no definite anterior wall or posterior myocardial infarction.

The patient had temporarily received procainamide for arrhythmia. When the condition deteriorated he was admitted to the hospital with severe pain in the back and arm, night sweats and a slight temperature and dyspnoea.

The patient received erythromycin for a suspected infection. Nevertheless, his general condition deteriorated and an intubation was performed.

An echocardiogram was not carried out – the patient was in an intensive care unit outside Europe.

There were various possibilities for the differential diagnosis. My suggestion was Lupus erythematosus. What was the basis for the pleural effusion? Procainamide can lead to such a syndrome. Neither does an allergy or a septic infection appear to be excluded.

What would you do about the dyspnoea? Who would administer nitroglycerin ex juvantibus?

One of the objectives of this discussion should be to point out that medications can also be used for *diagnostic* purposes. In situations where the diagnosis is not clear, a pharmaceutical can be temporarily administered and the reaction observed. Within several hours it is possible to determine if the heart is functioning better; the preload is reduced and therefore the overal heart function is improved. This "test" is performed far too rarely. Professor Bussmann demonstrated that following the administration of nitroglycerin the filling pressure sank considerably; from 50 to about 17 mmHg.

Hetzer: I think that it is a little early to infuse nitroglycerin without any further diagnostics.

Hugenholtz: Professor Hetzer, I beg to differ. What would you suggest? A pleurapunction indicated no evidence of an effusion. Nitroglycerin can certainly have a negative effect on the cardiac function; if the preload is lowered too much and thereby the output is reduced too far. This is not, however, true in the case of a backward failure. Of course an echocardiogram and then a punction would first of all be performed. Neither one of these were performed. Please keep in mind that this was a non-European clinic. Besides that, there was a functional tricuspidal insufficiency.

Auditorium: The configuration of the heart in the x-ray is definitely not typical for an acute heart insufficiency with effusion. In an emergency room it is often 30 to 60 minutes before an echo is available. Nitroglycerin on the other hand reduces the pressure immediately, indicates a diagnosis and directly helps the patient.

Hugenholtz: Professor Hetzer, you have optimal conditions in your clinic, an echocardiograph, transportation possibilities, assistants... In most parts of the world they have to get by with considerably less. Intensive care units do not even have an echocardiograph. What would you do under such conditions?

Hetzer: Other than the ambiguous x-ray, we hardly have any objective findings. It could be an embolism of the pulmonary artery, pneumonia or a number of differential diagnosis. And nitroglycerin should be administered in this situation? I don't agree with this "diagnostic test".

May I remind you about another diagnostic method? Is there an occlusion of the jugular? Even if there is no 2 D-echocardiograph available, there is at least a "normal" ultrasound device. If this is not available then it should at least be possible in an intensive care unit to install an atrial catheter or a pulmonary arterial catheter, which would supply important data on the hemodynamics. It does not appear acceptable to me to administer nitroglycerin before these examinations.

Hugenholtz: You said something important about the Swan-Ganz catheter. I agree with its use, whereby a therapeutic "test" is then possible? Do you insist, as does Professor Hetzer, that an echocardiograph must first of all be performed?

Auditorium: One wishes to know as soon as possible whether nitroglycerin is helping or causing harm. The registration of the blood pressure offers sufficient information as to whether it is right or not. This can be done in every hospital.

Bussmann: Thus far we have not paid any attention to a possible respiratory insufficiency. It has been emphasized that there are respiratory complains, that there is even a resting dyspnoea. Therefore a (pulmonary-caused) pulmonary edema can be assumed. In such a case I would indeed apply nitroglycerin sublingually. If this leads to improvement then you know that you are dealing with a left ventricular failure and therefore have made the proper diagnosis.

Hugenholtz: What importance does the role of the i. v. play in the administration of the nitroglycerin? There is certainly complete agreement with its use when the diagnosis is clear. In any case we would first of all apply the nitroglycerin ex juvantibus.

Auditorium: I have also treated such cases of partial ventricular insufficiency without manifested pulmonary edema where the blood pressure dropped to 90 mmHg for some time. There were then considerable breathing difficulties, but no heart failure.

Hugenholtz: In any case, this man was admitted to an intensive care unit and intubated. His condition improved. Two weeks later he was transferred to the general ward. He did however, continue to exhibit a cardiomegaly, pulmonary lung rales and effusion. The echo showed an ejection fraction of 35%. There were still edemas, some of which were on the leg where the surgeons had removed the bypass. Bleeding continued to manifest itself. This bleeding was based on a thrombocytopenia and originally attributable to a Lupus erythematodes visceralis.

The patient's condition improved slowly. Assuming a cardiac insufficiency erythromycin, captropil were administered; and steroids due to the Lupus – there were temporary arthritic complaints.

Was it as case of cardiac insufficiency, a general infection or a Lupus erythematodes with pneumonia, or was there an error in the therapy, the patient not recovering despite intensive efforts?

Hetzer: It is possible that a recurring pulmonary arterial embolism was the cause, because there were infiltrations on the left.

Hugenholtz: Pulmonary embolism – are there other suggestions? Thrombopenia and tendency to bleed continued to be present.

Hetzer: Was the procainamide treatment temporarily interrupted?

Hugenholtz: Procainamide was stopped; it is, however possible that this should have happened earlier. It is often noted that in practice physicians do not treat the illness or the cause, but rather the symptoms. The arrhythmia, which was treated for months with procainamide, did not have anything to with the primary disease – Lupus erythematodes.

O'Rourke: Was HIV detected?

Hugenholtz: Not that I am aware.

O'Rourke: In view of the previous blood transfusions and the severe pneumonia, that is not misleading.

Hugenholtz: Do the symptoms described indicate AIDS? It could very well have been a case of pneumocystis-carinii-pneumonia.

Jugdutt: At first I thought of cardiac insufficiency or an aorta dissection because of the back pain. It could also be an inferior mycardial infarction with right and left ventricular involvement.

Hetzer: In my opinion everything points to the Lupus erythematodes, whereby I would administer more than 42 mg steroids. The renal function is also inhibited, meaning it could be a quickly progressing Lupus. I would administer higher dosages of steroids or cyclophosphamide. When all else fails a plasmapheresis could be considered.

Bussmann: The patient obviously has a pleura effusion and pulmonary infiltration at various locations, at present mainly on the left, previously on the right. The patient has been bedridden for some time with a relapsing pneumonia. It could be a "plain old" cardiac insufficiency.

Hugenholtz: Then we should intensify our therapy. Up to now we have only administered captopril. What do you think of nitrates?

Bussmann: Have diuretics been used? We have to try to exclude Lupus erythematodes which would be connected with operative therapy. If a heart insufficiency with pleura exudation is assumed, the cardiac function has to be checked – so why not apply nitroglycerin?

Hugenholtz: That is exactly what I wanted to hear! I can now offer you a solution to the puzzle. The patient died in a coma. Here are the six aortocoronary bypasses. One of them is open at the anterior descending artery, another, which supplies the posterior wall, is completely occluded. The others are open, but stenosized.

Furthermore, new infarctions, a clearly hypertrophic, fibrotic heart and arteriosclerotic plaque in the coronary vessels were detected. Do you think that such a radically altered heart would react at all to nitrates or that nitroglycerin is the proper therapy?

Hetzer: It was not correct to perform sequential bypasses. Three such bypasses were done. Today we know that the occlusion rate of such bypasses is much higher than with single bypasses.

Hugenholtz: The operation was performed six years ago.

Hetzer: We would have reoperated.

Hugenholtz: Here you see the lungs. The pathologists described this as a chronic blood stasis with cardiac insufficiency. What then is the diagnosis?

Aspergillos-mycosis of the lungs! That was not discovered in the course of two months

Auditorium: In view of the findings established at the beginning of the illness (x-ray with enlarged heart, pleura exudation on the right side, temperatures) not enough was done to make a diagnosis.

Hugenholtz: Cultures from the sputum and the pleurapunction did not propagate. Too much effort was attached to the Lupus erythematodes and related the infection to the illness as well as the various Lupus factors, ANF.

Hetzer: We have also often lost patients in which aspergillos was detected in the post mortem. A very good mycologic institute exists in Berlin. Nowadays we see aspergillos more often than in the past, but we still have difficulties with the diagnosis. The number of undiagnosed cases appears to be larger.

Hugenholtz: A fungal pneumonia still appears to have a specific set of prerequisites, for example an extended stay in intensive care. Furtermore, this patient suffered a severe coronary disease, whereby almost all of the coronary arteries were completely occluded. This, and the treatment with antibiotics, had evidently promoted the growth of the fungus.

The greatest instrument in all of medicine is the retrospectoscope. In this case it was used to diagnose aspergillosis, which is much more prominent and has to be diagnosed much earlier than presently is done.

Awarding of the Nitrolingual Prize 1990

Athur Boskamp: Dr. Münzel has been chosen to receive the prize.

The work is entitled:

"Nitrate tolerance in epicardial arteries or in the venous system is not reversed by N-acetylcysteine in vivo, but tolerance-independent interactions exist"

With this investigation, Dr. Münzel counters an assumption of nitrate tolerance which claims that intracellular SH-group loading would be exhausted by the prolonged effect of nitrates, and that this memory could be refilled by an SH-group supplier such as N-acetylcysteine. Dr. Münzel's results now show that N-acetylcysteine has no influence on nitrate tolerance, but rather produces only a general enhancement of nitrate effect.

As has recently been learned, the regulation mechanisms in blood vessels are highly dependent on the endothelium and can in a similar way also be influenced by nitroglycerin; they are, therefore, not so easily represented.

Continued research on this topic, based on Dr. Münzel's analyses, is most welcome.

For now, though, I would like to move on to the actual award.

Congratulations, Dr. Münzel. First the memorial medal, then your certificate as recipient of the Nitrolingual Prize. Again, congratulations and our best wishes.

Dr. Münzel: I would like to express my sincere thanks for this prize and perhaps briefly point out the clinical implications of this experiment, although it was conducted on animals. Our problem before 1987 was that Becker had shown that tolerance can be modified with N-acetylcysteine, yet only partially lifted. I believe at this point, many people called up Pohl-Boskamp to ask "How much N-acetylcysteine has to be administered in order to offset a tolerance development?"

Our findings fit quite well into the concept, which was also presented by Mr. Noack. Microcirculation can not biologically transform glyceroltrinitrate. No NO can be stored. If we allow for high doses of N-acetylcysteine, the separation of the NO radical from NO is improved; yet in effect, this again results in resistant vessel effcct, which is tolerance-independent and, in our opinion, has nothing to do with a specific lifting of nitrate tolerance by intracellular mechanisms.

Bei Fragen zur Produktsicherheit wenden Sie sich bitte an:
If you have any questions regarding product safety,
please contact:

Walter de Gruyter GmbH
Genthiner Straße 13
10785 Berlin
productsafety@degruyterbrill.com